DISEASES AND PARASITES OF POULTRY

DISEASES AND PARASITES OF POULTRY

Editor
Gove Hambidge

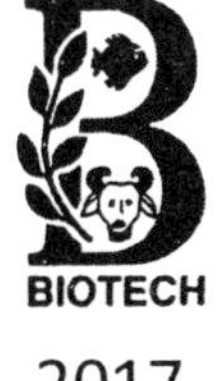

2017
Biotech Books

ISBN10 81-7622-088-4
ISBN13 978-81-7622-088-0
EAN 9788176220880

Original Title: Livestock Yearbook of Agriculture, 1942

Published by : **BIOTECH BOOKS**
1123/74, Tri Nagar,
Delhi - 110 035
Phone: 27109765
e-mail: biotechbooks@yahoo.co.in

Showroom : 4762-63/23, Ansari Road, Darya Ganj,
New Delhi - 110 002
Phone: 23245578, 23244987

Laser Typesetting : **Classic Computer Services**
Delhi - 110 035

Printed at : **Chawla Offset Printers**
Delhi - 110 052

PRINTED IN INDIA

CONTENTS

INTRODUCTION

Pullorum Disease

The poison-forming germ, *Salmonella pullorum*, primarily attacks the ovaries in hens and may produce no visible symptoms or signs except reduced productivity of the hen and hatchability of its eggs. In chicks, however, it produces a devastating disease, formerly called bacillary white diarrhoea, which may practically exterminate an entire brood within three weeks after hatching. The germ is transmitted through the egg and also in excreta and on bits of contaminated material, such as fluff, floating in the air. The disease is extremely contagious and infectious. Unfortunately, many of the infected chicks do not die but grow up and in their turn produce infected eggs, perpetuating and spreading the malady. Thus pullorum disease has become exceptionally widespread and has been responsible for enormous losses to poultrymen. It is one of the major problems of the hatchery industry, since a few infected eggs in one of the giant modern incubators are a source of danger to the whole hatch.

There is no medicinal cure or preventive for pullorum disease and control depends fundamentally on locating and eliminating all carrier hens. Agglutination tests have been developed that make this possible. Three methods are commonly used, all involving expert skill and labouratory facilities. Bunyea describes them with a degree of detail that gives the layman an insight into the kind of procedures involved in making tests for various diseases.

1. The long method, or tube test, involves taking samples of blood from fowl and sending them in test tubes packed in ice to a labouratory, where the blood serum is mixed with a specially prepared suspension of bacteria, known as an

antigen, derived from cultures of the pullorum germ. In a positive reaction, the bacteria are clumped together and settle to the bottom of the tube, leaving the fluid clear. This method is relatively costly and the other two have been developed in recent years to reduce the expense of testing and bring it within reach of more poultrymen.

2. In the rapid serum test the serum from the blood of the fowl is mixed with a concentrated antigen on a glass plate over an illuminated dark background. In a positive test the bacteria are clumped together and separate in the form of particles or masses that are easily visible, with clear surrounding fluid, whereas in a negative reaction the smear remains uniformly cloudy.
3. The stained antigen, rapid whole-blood test, the most recently developed method, does not require the collection of serum and it can be carried out on the farm. A single drop of blood is mixed with a single drop of antigen, which has been stained with crystal violet, on a white glass plate. In a positive test, the stained bacteria clump together and are easily seen as violet-coloured particles.

With these tests as a weapon and the seriousness of the disease as a motive, a National Poultry Improvement Plan was inaugurated in 1935 to make a concerted drive against the scourge on a countrywide scale. The plan is administered by State officials cooperating with the Federal Bureau of Animal Industry. By 1940-41, 44 States were participating and nearly 9 million birds had been tested. Under the plan, flocks are certified in three classes, U.S. Pullorum-Tested, U.S. Pullorum-Passed and U.S. Pullorum-Clean.

Reports from all over the country indicate that as a result of this plan, the hatchability of eggs is improving and the mortality among chicks decreasing.

Meanwhile pullorum disease has become increasingly important as a menace to the turkey industry. Turkey poults seem to be very susceptible and suffer a high mortality. The tests used for chickens do not give as clear-cut results with turkeys and more work is being done on this problem. The best preventive is to have turkey hatching and brooding done entirely separate from these operations with chickens.

Fowl Paralysis and Other Forms of the Avian Leukosis Complex

Of the $100,000,00 toll taken by poultry diseases every year in the United States alone, about half is due to a disease, or a group of diseases, concerning which science knows comparatively little. The manifestation of this disease complex most familiar to poultrymen is probably fowl paralysis, also called range paralysis, in which the nerves are affected so that the bird is partly or completely paralysed. But there are many other manifestations described in this article by Brandly, Waters and Hall. One type affects the eye, causing loss of colour in the iris, bulging of the eyeball, changes in the size and shape of the pupil and sometimes partial or total blindness. Another, the visceral type, affects the internal organs–liver, lungs, heart, spleen, ovary, testicles, kidneys, intestines–causing loss of flesh, weakness and non-productiveness. In still another type, the long bones become thickened and enlarged. In the blood type, there are alterations in the blood, the circulation and sometimes the bone marrow (source of red blood cells) which may quickly endanger the life of the bird. A dozen or more lengthy scientific names have been applied to these various manifestations, all of which have features that are similar and also are suggestive of certain diseases of other animals and human beings.

Fowl paralysis first appeared in this country about 1920 and in the twenty-odd years since, there has been a good deal of scattered investigation of the avian leukosis complex. Quite recently, in 1938, a Regional Poultry Research Labouratory was established by the United States Department of Agriculture at East Lansing, Mich. and here major attention is being given to this disease group. The work of the labouratory is done in co-operation with 25 States in the North Central and Northeastern States.

What is the cause of the disease complex and how is it spread? No one yet knows. Apparently poor nutrition, an unfavourable environment and parasitic infestation are not causes, though any of them may well predispose birds to attack. Nor have any specific bacteria been found to cause the disease. Most authorities consider that a virus or viruslike agent is responsible. Various types of the disease can be transmitted by inoculating young birds with material prepared from the blood or organs of diseased birds, but how it is transmitted under ordinary conditions has not been discovered.

There are indications that it is passed on through the egg and also by contact. Resistance increases rather rapidly with age and apparently there are inherited differences in susceptibility. All in all, pending further knowledge, the best practical advice that can be given to poultrymen for combating this malady is to use strict sanitary measures in the whole process of raising poultry and to follow careful breeding procedures, mating only birds from blood lines that have a record of good health and high viability and closing flocks to outside breeding.

The authors of this article review much of the scientific work that has been done to date on the avian leukosis complex and then describe in some detail the coordinated investigations being carried on at the regional labouratory. In these investigations, genetics and pathology are receiving major attention at first. Because of the lack of knowledge about the cause of the disease and how it spreads, the physical arrangements at the labouratory involve extraordinary precautions to prevent un-intentional transmission of the disease from one group of birds to another.

In the genetic work an effort is being made to form families inherently resistant and families inherently susceptible to the avian leukosis complex, the latter to be used in pathological studies and also in determining the mode of inheritance of resistance and the influence of the environment. Ten different White Leghorn strains are being used. The pathology programme includes studies on methods of diagnosis, means of detecting carriers, means of transmission, nature and tissue distribution of the causative agent, embryo and chick susceptibility and the mechanism of acquired immunity, Several strains of the avian leukosis complex are being used in inoculation experiments. Other aspects of the problem that will need to be studied include management, nutritional and physiological factors.

Respiratory Diseases of Chickens and Turkeys

Hall discusses a group of diseases that cause heavy losses in flocks throughout the country, especially in winter, when replacement is costly.

Infectious laryngotracheitis, a virus disease, comes on suddenly and in an acute form may be fatal in loss than a week; a less virulent attack may last 3 weeks. Mortality may be as high as 70 per cent and the disease also causes a marked drop in egg production. The outstanding symptoms are gasping and coughing, caused by the collection of mucus, pus and blood in the respiratory passages. Diagnosis is not easy because of possible confusion with other respiratory diseases; a labouratory diagnostic test may be necessary. A bird that recovers naturally from the disease becomes a carrier for life and these carriers are the principal spreaders of the virus. Strict sanitation and vaccination are the best preventives. The vaccine is applied to the mucous membrane of the cloaca by scarifying with a stiff bristle brush. Immunity lasts for the life of the bird. Hall says that vaccination should not be practiced if the disease does not exist in the neighbourhood and there is little or no chance that the flock will be exposed to it.

Infectious bronchitis, probably also caused by a virus, is primarily a disease of young chicks. Mortality ranges from 10 to 90 percent. As in laryngotracheitis, diagnosis is difficult and labouratory tests may be necessary. Vaccination is not practicable because the virus in the vaccine reaches the lungs before immunity is established. The best preventives are careful inspection of purchased chicks, good management of brooder houses, thorough disinfection after an outbreak of the disease.

Infectious fowl coryza (coryza is the medical term for a cold) is an acute inflammatory contagious disease primarily affecting the upper air passages, sinuses and eye membranes. It occurs in two types, a very rapid one, caused by a germ and a slower one, of which the cause is not definitely known. (Fowl cholera can also cause a coryza.) The first symptom is a watery discharge from the nasal passages and often the eyes; later symptoms may be severe. A bacteriological examination and labouratory tests may be necessary for a definite diagnosis. Just how the disease spreads is not known. Preventives include careful attention to housing conditions and nutrition; in California, where "colds" occur annually among pullets, disposal or segregation of old stock before pullets are brought in is recommended. Recently it has been found that sulphathiazole is effective in the treatment of the germ-produced, acute type of coryza.

Non-infectious coryzas may also be caused by a vitamin A deficiency (nutritional roup) and by mechanical irritation. The former is cured by adding supplements rich in vitamin A to the diet.

Sinusitis in turkeys, also called roup and swellhead, is a coryza characterized by swelling of the sinuses in front of the eyes. It may be infectious (cause unknown) or nutritional. The infectious type may be treated successfully by injections of argyrol or silver nitrate according to procedures described by Hall. The nutritional type may be prevented by furnishing an adequate amount of vitamin A in the diet.

Fowl Pox (Diphtheria)

It used to be thought, says Bunyea, that fowl pox and avian diphtheria were two separate diseases. Now it is known that they are different manifestations of a single disease, caused by a virus. In the pox form; characterized by the formation of blisters and later scabs on the skin–usually are unfeathered parts–the disease is generally mild. The diphtheritic form, in which cheesy patches appear on the mucous membranes of the mouth, air passages and eyes, interfering with breathing and eating, may be fatal. Recovery from the disease confers a prolonged immunity. The virus enters the body through scratches or wounds in the skin or mucous membranes and dried material from diseased birds remains infectious for a long time.

There are two types or strains of the virus. One produces the symptoms in pigeons; the other affects all other fowl. Pigeons are relatively resistant to the fowl type and other fowl to the pigeon type.

Poultry can be successfully vaccinated against fowl pox with vaccines prepared from either type of virus. The usual procedure is to apply the vaccine with a stiff bristle brush to feather follicles on a prepared area of skin, or to stab it into the skin with needles; if pigeon pox vaccine is used for chickens, 12 to 20 feather follicles are inoculated instead of only a few, as when fowl pox vaccine is used. The vaccine, which was formerly prepared from pox scabs, is now prepared from virus propagated on developing chick embryos. Vaccination of healthy birds after an outbreak occurs is worth while only if the disease is in a mild form and if the vaccinating is done early, in the outbreak.

There is no known cure for fowl pox and if an outbreak is severe or has been prolonged, it is best to slaughter affected birds. If they are exceptionally valuable, they may be kept under quarantine to await possible recovery. In any event, as soon as the disease appears, the affected and the healthy birds should be separated and strict sanitary measures, including disinfection of quarters from which diseased birds are removed, should be put into effect. Poultry keepers should be on their guard against introduction of the disease into pox-free flocks or areas.

Psittacosis

The striking new development disclosed by Meyer is that a case of psittacosis (so-called parrot fever) in a human being has apparently been traced to chickens and 10 other cases have been traced to pigeons.

Psittacosis was first discovered as a disease of birds of the parrot family and occasionally of other cage birds such as canaries and finches. The fact that it causes a peculiar type of pneumonia in human beings, reputed to be fatal in 20 percent of the cases, has been known for a long time; but human psittacosis was a medical curiosity until over 750 cases occurred in 1929-30 and 600 more were recorded in subsequent years. As a result, embargoes on imported birds and other restrictive measures were put into effect in the United States. Some States maintain a permanent quarantine against birds of the parrot family. In an effort to stamp out the disease, California has instituted a system, described by Meyer, requiring testing of parrakeets in commercial a viaries and certification of the aviary.

Psittacosis is caused by a virus and is highly infective; it can be spread, for instance, by particles of dust floating in the air. It can now be diagnosed by a blood test and also by an inoculation test with mice, which are very susceptible. These methods have been extremely useful in detecting carriers–apparently healthy birds that harbour and disseminate the virus.

A few years ago it was proved by experiment that chickens are susceptible to the disease. Subsequently, a fatal case of human psittacosis was traced to a sick pigeon; then 9 other cases were traced to pigeons; and finally tests made to pigeon flocks in 5 States showed a surprisingly high percentage of positive reactions. The most recent discovery, already noted, was the isolation of the virus from 2 chickens on a poultry farm in the course of an investigation of a human case of the disease. It has also been isolated from 25 individual pigeons.

How widespread is the infection among birds on farms? How do they acquire it? What is the risk to human beings? These, as Meyer points out, are among the pressing questions posed by the new discoveries.

Miscellaneous Diseases of Poultry

Bunyea covers a number of diseases, most of which are not discussed elsewhere in the section devoted to poultry.

Paratyphoid infection, caused by organisms of the *Salmonella* group, occurs mainly in young birds, may be either acute or chronic and has various symptoms. It is difficult to control; sanitation in hatching and rearing the young is of first importance. Both infected duck eggs and the flesh of infected squabs may cause food poisoning in human beings, but possible danger from this source is eliminated if these products are thoroughly cooked.

Fowl typhoid, like fowl cholera, is caused by bacteria that live in the blood stream. No remedy or vaccine is available; sanitary measures are important in preventing the disease. The blood test for pullorum disease also detects typhoid carriers. Fowl typhoid is detecting among chickens, increasing among turkeys.

Fowl cholera, characterized by intestinal disturbances, depression and mortality, may be either acute or chronic. Fortunately the bacteria are easily destroyed by sanitary measures. A rapid wholeblood test for the diagnosis of fowl cholera carriers is a recent development. Although not yet widely used, it is a possible aid in detecting the birds that are harbouring the infection.

Mycosis includes three types of disease due to different fungi:

(1) Thrush is due to the presence of fungi in the digestive tract. It produces a discharge from the mouth, loss of appetite, weakness, emaciation and diarrhoea and is frequently fatal. Thorough sanitation is the best preventive, but Bunyea also describes a simple medicinal treatment.

(2) Aspergillosis is caused by fungi in the air passages. It produces gasping, unthriftiness and emaciation and may easily be confused with other respiratory diseases. In young

chicks it is rapidly fatal. Strict sanitation is the only known preventive. Sick birds should be segregated or destroyed.

(3) Favus (white comb, avian mycotic dermatitis) is caused by a fungus that attacks the skill. Growths or crusts appear on the unfeathered head parts; elsewhere feathers break off. The disease is said to infect human beings. Treatment with petroleum jelly and formalin, as described by Bunyea, is reported to be very effective.

Infectious avian encephalomyelitis (epidemic tremor), an inflammation of the central nervous system, is spread by direct contact and may be passed on through the egg. A large percentage of a flock may be affected. Although spontaneous recoveries occur, it is recommended that infected birds be quickly fattened and marketed to eliminate carriers.

Avian tuberculosis is discussed in the general article on tuberculosis in this volume. A few additional points are given by Bunyea.

Poisoning of poultry may be due to various causes:

(1) Botulism (limber-neck) is caused by eating feed or other products contaminated with the botulinus organism and its toxins. The condition is likely to be rapidly fatal. Exposed birds may be drenched with Epsom salts and given antitoxin injections.

(2) Common sources of chemical poisoning of poultry include rat poisons, vegetation sprayed with arsenicals, fish brine, ice-cream salt, spent fireworks, poisoned grasshoppers and grasshopper bait and certain worm medicines.

(3) Even small numbers of the insects known as rose chafers will poison young chickens.

Lameness may also be due to anyone of various causes:

(1) Wire cloth with a large mesh may catch the feet or legs of chicks.

(2) Toes and feet may be frozen in cold weather if the birds are not kept in properly arranged houses.

(3) Bumblefoot, a swelling characterized by an accumulation of cheesy material, is probably due to infection of wounds.

It causes great suffering and should be treated by minor surgery, disinfection and bandaging.

(4) Sod disease is an inflammation of the skin accompanied by small swellings filled with fluid. It may affect the feet and the eyelids and is often fatal. The cause is unknown, but birds should be excluded from unplowed prairie land.

(5) Nutritional deficiencies, discussed elsewhere in this volume, may cause lameness.

(6) Fowl paralysis, also discussed elsewhere, is manifested in lameness. Avian tuberculosis, paratyphoid infection and fowl cholera may all cause lameness. Infection with one of the staphylococcus organisms is responsible for a lameness in the feet, legs or wings that often ends in death.

(7) Scaly leg, discussed in the article on poultry mites, is a condition caused by a parasitic itch mite.

"It is normal for a fowl to be in good condition if it is given a chance," says Bunyea. He discusses some of the practices that give the birds such a chance, among them:

(1) Proper location of the poultry house.

(2) Clean, comfortable, well-ventilated houses; abundant, nourishing feed; clean water.

(3) Proper management of brooder houses.

(4) Frequent moving of houses or shelters for growing birds on the range to keep the birds off polluted ground.

(5) Cleaned, disinfected, dry laying houses ready for the birds when they come off the range.

(6) Separate houses for pullets and old hens and for birds of different species.

(7) Mesh wire, or preferably fly screening, on doors and windows.

(8) Exclusion of all visitors from the poultry houses; provision of clean overshoes for those admitted; disinfection of the soles of footwear when entering the poultry house if certain diseases are prevalent in the area.

(9) Quarantining of newly purchased birds or those that have returned from contests or shows.

(10) Prompt action in cases of infectious diseases, including destruction or segregation of sick birds and disinfection of premises.

Internal Parasites of Poultry

Chickens are kept on 85 percent of the farms of the United States, which makes it all the more striking that almost a fifth of the birds are lost every year because of disease. The annual financial loss has been estimated at 180 million dollars, a good deal of it waste because it is preventable.

Wehr and Christensen describe the practices necessary to reduce the part of this loss that is due to internal parasites. These practices depend chiefly on three simple facts:

(1) Most, though not all, poultry parasites are eliminated in the droppings of the birds.

(2) In the crowded poultry communities of today, the surroundings quickly become contaminated.

(3) Birds pick up parasites from these contaminated surroundings–feed, water, soil and infected intermediate hosts such as snails and slugs.

The great preventive, then, is to have clean surroundings. This means, for example, carefully selecting the site for the poultry house; using a type of house that can easily be kept clean; not crowding the birds in runs or yards that cannot be kept clean–instead, either using a series of runs that can be rotated, or confining the birds entirely within the house except perhaps for a "porch" with a wire floor or a small fenced yard covered with cinders or other porous material; disposing of manure promptly and storing it properly; keeping different types of poultry, such as turkeys and chickens or turkeys and pigeons, entirely separate, since a disease that is mild for one type may be disastrous for another and being careful not to spread infection on shoes or clothing. Following these general principles of good hygiene and at the same time feeding the birds well will go a long way toward preventing trouble with parasites.

If an outbreak of parasitism occurs, the healthy birds and the diseased birds should be promptly separated and kept separate and a strict sanitation programme should be carried out. If no local veterinarian is available to make a diagnosis and advise on treatment, the State Agricultural Experiment Station should be consulted as to the advisability of sending birds to the labouratory for diagnosis.

There is little in the way of medicinal treatment for most poultry parasites, the authors point out, through anthelmintics, or worm medicines, are effective for the gapeworm, the large roundworm and the cecum worm; and trichomoniasis of the lower digestive tract of turkeys can be successfully treated by heat therapy–closing the birds for certain periods of time in a box heated to a certain temperature.

After discussing these practical control measures, the authors deal in considerable detail with the principal poultry parasites.

With the exception of coccidiosis, discussed elsewhere in this volume, the diseases produced by protozoa are important mainly in turkeys.

A severe catarrhal inflammation of the intestines of turkeys, caused by a protozoan called *Hexamita meleagridis*, is becoming increasingly important in the United States. The mortality in acute outbreaks runs from 20 to 90 percent and most birds that recover from an acute attack remain stunted. Adult turkeys are the primary source of infection.

Histomoniasis, or so-called blackhead (the head does not always; turn dark), is an acute, highly fatal disease caused by infection with *Histomonas meleagridis*. Until methods of preventing it, based on sanitation, were found, this disease made turkey raising impossible in many parts of the country. Chickens, which are not seriously affected by histomoniasis, become carriers; so do the few turkeys that recover.

A malaria like disease of young turkey poults and ducklings is caused by organisms of the genus *Leucocytozoon*, which attack the blood cells. The disease strikes suddenly in young birds and runs a brief, acute course, with a mortality up to 50 percent in turkeys and 100 percent in ducklings. The causative organisms are transmitted by blackflies.

Two species of trichomonads cause intestinal disturbances in young turkeys, one attacking the crop and gullet the other the cecum and liver. Occasionally, though not usually, the mortality from trichomoniasis of the upper digestive tract is high. The disease in the lower digestive tract may be confused with histomoniasis and often takes an insidious, slow course, ending in death.

A considerable number of worm parasites of the general types that attack other animals, are found in poultry.

At least three species of flukes, or trematodes, parasitize poultry, but none are of great economic importance. One occurs in the skin of domestic and wild birds, producing hard, cystlike structures, usually in the region of the vent. Another, found in muskrats and water birds, may be responsible for an inflammation of the proventriculus, or true stomach, in chickens. A third is located in the reproductive organs and can greatly reduce or completely stop egg production in laying hens, as well as causing extreme emaciation and anemia. Snails and dragonflies are the intermediate hosts of this fluke.

Several species of tapeworms (cestodes) inhabit the small intestines of fowl; all pass through certain stages of development, when they are known as bladder worms, in intermediate hosts, including houseflies, snails, slugs, ants, earthworms, beetles grasshoppers and sandhoppers. Fowl become infected by swallowing the intermediate hosts.

Roundworms, or nematodes, which parasitize almost every organ in the body of birds, include three groups–those that are transmitted directly, those that are transmitted through intermediate hosts such as various insects and those that are transmitted in both ways. Among the nematodes are the crop worms, the stomach worms, the gizzard worms, the large intestinal roundworms, the small intestinal roundworms, the eye worm and gapeworms, which infest the windpipe and cause the condition known as gapes. The nematodes cause more or less severe illness and sometimes death, depending on the severity of the infestation. In the case of *Ascaridia galli*, one of the large intestinal roundworms, it has been shown that foods high in vitamin A and in the B vitamins increase resistance and that a lack of the vitamin B complex definitely favors parasitism.

Coccidiosis of the Chicken

Coccidiosis occurs in all domesticated fowl and in cattle, sheep, goats, pigs and dogs, but, as Christensen and Allen point out, it probably causes heavier economic losses among chickens than among all the rest combined.

The life history of the common coccidia of poultry goes like this:

(1) The egg like, resistant oöcysts are discharged in the birds' droppings.

(2) Each oöcyst divides into four elongated bodies and each of these into two sporozoites.

(3) An oöcyst thus divided (sporulated) is swallowed by a chicken.

(4) The eight sporozoites are released in the intestinal canal and penetrate cells in the membrane tissue.

(5) After growth, each divides into many merozoites, which parasitize other cells.

(6) Again growth and division occur.

(7) Finally, some of the merozoites develop into males and females and mate.

(8) The fertilized females secrete a resistant shell, becoming oöcysts and are discharged in the droppings.

Coccidia may become localized in the cecum, causing an acute, often highly fatal disease, mostly of chicks 3 to 5 weeks old, characterized by severe cecal hemorrhage; or they may become localized mainly in the small intestine, causing a serious, prolonged disease of older birds characterized by extreme emaciation. The first disease is caused by *Eimeria tenella*, the second by any one of at least six species of coccidia, of which *Eimeria necatrix* produces the most severe symptoms.

In addition to the deaths caused by coccidiosis, many of the birds that recover are permanently unthrifty, as well as being carriers of the infection.

Control of the disease consists in strict isolation .of young birds from adult fowl and in extremely careful sanitation, including such measures as thorough, regular, frequent cleaning of brooder houses with soap and hot water; daily cleaning of chick cages; frequent cleaning of feeding and watering equipment; occasional transfer of movable brooder houses to new ground; careful locating of permanent brooder houses and provision of sloping concrete runs; the same kind of cleaning of laying houses as of brooder houses; provision of clean ground for each group of pullets.

In case of an outbreak, medication does little good, but losses can be minimized by meticulous attention to every detail of good feeding and care.

Poultry Lice and their Control

All the lice that attack poultry, says Bishopp, are of the biting and chewing rather than the bloodsucking type. They cause heavy indirect losses, probably chiefly among farm and backyard flocks. The specialized poultry keeper usually does not permit them to get a foothold and there is no reason why they should not be controlled even in the smallest flock.

All lice live continuously on the host and soon die if removed, but different kinds attack different parts of the body.

The head louse is usually found on the top and back of the head and beneath the bill. Among lice, it is the chief pest of young chickens and turkeys, sometimes causing death before the birds are a month old. The body louse of chickens stays on the skin, usually where the body is not densely feathered and is the most important of the lice attacking adult birds. The shaft louse rests on the shafts of the feathers and apparently feeds only on feathers. Four other fairly common chicken lice are the wing louse, the fluff louse, the large chicken louse and the brown chicken louse.

Turkeys are subject to the attacks of the slender turkey louse and the large turkey louse, as well as of chicken lice. Geese and ducks are seldom noticeably affected by lice, but there are six species that attack pigeons, sometimes damaging the feathers of show birds and perhaps adversely affecting the speed and endurance of carriers.

In general it is best to delouse the poultry flock in the fall so that they will be free of these pests through the following spring. Treatment with sodium fluoride is very effective and practical. Each bird may be thoroughly dusted (most expensive method); or the insecticide may be applied in small pinches to several designated parts of the body; or the birds may be dipped in a solution containing 1 table-spoonful of sodium fluoride to each gallon of water (least expensive method). Sodium fluoride irritates the air passages when breathed in and is a poison when taken internally and Bishopp outlines the necessary precautions in handling it. Sodium fluosilicate may also be used as a dip. Other treatments, not so effective, are the use of fine sulfur as a dust and the painting of roosts with nicotine sulfate.

Poultry Mites

A large percentage of poultry of all kinds, according to Bishopp, are constantly infested with mites which lower the vitality of the birds, reduce their egg production and in some cases actually cause death.

The common chicken mite is what Bishopp calls a night raider, generally hiding in cracks and crevices during the day. It attacks all parts of the body and feeds by sucking blood and it will attack other animals and human beings as well as poultry. Heavily infested setting hens have been known to die on the nest. To get rid of these mites, remove all boards, boxes and trash that might serve as hiding places; burn the litter and nesting material; spray the poultry house thoroughly with one of the carbolineums, crude petroleum, or creosote oil. One treatment is usually enough.

The feather mite, which remains constantly on the birds, requires a different treatment. Each bird should be dipped in a sulfur bath (2 ounces of fine sulfur and 1 ounce of soap to a gallon of water) on a warm, sunny day or in a heated building; or the birds may be thoroughly dusted with sulfur; or nicotine sulfate may be applied to the perches. The house should also be disinfected as for the common chicken mite.

The scaly-leg mite attacks the shanks and feet and sometimes the comb, wattles and neck. The legs of infested birds may be dipped in crude petroleum. Painting the roosts and nests with a carbolineum also helps to control this mite.

The depluming mite burrows in the skin near the base of the feathers. It may be completely eliminated by dipping each bird in the sulfur bath already described.

Chiggers, the young of the small red harvest mite, attack chickens as well as other animals and human beings. They inject an irritating poison into the skin, to which they attach themselves (they do not burrow in as is commonly supposed). Severe infestations can have a very serious effect on young chickens and turkeys; hence in chigger areas it is best to hatch early or keep. the chicks from late hatches out of grass and weeds. Dusting the birds and the ranges with sulfur is helpful.

The Fowl Tick

The fowl tick, or blue bug, is a serious handicap to poultry raising in the Southwest, Bishopp points out and it now also occurs in Florida. Its attacks weaken the birds and cause a tick paralysis; egg production is reduced and not in frequently the birds die.

The tick, a flat, oval, leathery-skinned creature, resists many insecticides and can live for more than 3 years without food. It feeds exclusively on blood, preferring birds but also occasionally attacking domestic animals and human beings. Active at night, when the birds are on the roosts, it hides by day in cracks and crevices and is often shipped around the country concealed in poultry crates and other objects. In heavy infestations it may spread from poultry houses to barns and other buildings.

The tick can be controlled by thorough spraying of the building with one of the carbolineums; crude petroleum and creosote oil are less satisfactory. A second application 20 or 30 days after the first may be necessary and sometimes even a third. Bishopp gives directions for the spraying job. He also tells briefly how to construct roosts and nests to make control of the tick comparatively easy.

The fowl tick can be prevented from getting a foothold by such measures as proper choosing of a site and proper construction of a poultry house, buying chicks from tick-free hatcheries, thoroughly spraying used crates and isolating, for a period of 10 days, any fowl brought to the place.

Bedbugs as Pests of Poultry

Bedbugs are common pests of poultry as well as of human beings and domestic animals; in fact, as Back and Bishopp point out, they can easily be carried from poultry houses, where they hide in cracks and holes, to human dwellings. Wooden poultry crates are often heavily infested. The bugs feed mostly at night or in subdued light, take about two days to digest a full meal and can go without food for as long as 2 months. When they are abundant, they suck so much blood that chickens do not fatten and setting hens may die and the effects are especially disastrous in the case of squabs. The Mexican chicken bug (coruco, adobe bug), an important pest of poultry in the Southwest, is very much like the bedbug.

Keeping these insects under control requires vigilance and persistent effort. Hiding places should be eliminated as far as possible by simple construction, the removal of stray boards and trash and where it is practicable, the filling of cracks. Fumigants, such as burning sulfur, are effective in killing the bugs if the poultry house is tight enough (but few are). Thorough spraying with creosote oil or a carbolineum is satisfactory and so are kerosene and pyrethrum-kerosene fly sprays. In feeding establishments, it is well to spray crates once a month. In pigeon lofts, spraying the nests if not properly done may have a bad effect on eggs and squabs; treating the lofts with live steam has been effective under some circumstances.

The Pigeon Fly

A little smaller than a housefly and very active, the pigeon fly is a parasite only of pigeons and their close relatives. Bishopp describes how the insect crawls rapidly about among the feathers and sucks blood from both adult birds and squabs. In addition to causing irritation and loss of blood, it carries the pigeon malaria organism. It also bites human beings.

The fly lays neither eggs nor larvae, but pupae already formed, from which adult flies emerge, usually in about a month or less. These egg-shaped pupae tend to drop to the bottom of the nest boxes. The simplest way to control the pest, then, is to clean the nests and floors thoroughly every 25 days. The trash should be burned, or stored in a screened manure pit or bin equipped with a fly trap, or promptly spread and plowed under. Thorough soaking with a high-grade pyrethrum-kerosene spray will also kill the pupae

Adult flies on squabs can be killed by applying two or three pinches of pyrethrum, derris, or cube powder. Kerosene extract of pyrethrum kills the flies on adult birds or squabs and also in handling and killing rooms. When used on the birds, it should be applied with great care.

Once a loft has been freed of pigeon flies, Bishopp emphasizes, it should be kept free.

Nutritional Diseases of Poultry

Before discussing a considerable number of nutritional diseases of poultry, Titus points out that knowledge in this field is in a state of active change.

Vitamin A

Perhaps the primary function of vitamin A is the nourishment and repair of the epithelial structures (skin and internal membranes), which are the body's first line of defense against infection. It is also necessary for the normal functioning of the eye. In severe cases of deficiency, practically every organ of the body is affected. There are degenerative changes in the nerves and the eyes are inflamed. A partial deficiency in the diet of chickens, especially after dry weather has damaged green for age, is more common than is ordinarily supposed. Titus gives the amounts of vitamin A needed by chicks, turkey poults, chickens kept, for egg production and breeding stock and also, the amounts contained in the richer sources of this vitamin used in feeding.

Vitamin B_1

According to present evidence, vitamin B_1 is necessary for the proper metabolism of carbohydrates; in its absence, pyruvic acid, an intermediate product of this metabolism, accumulates and has a toxic effect on the nervous system. A deficiency does not occur in ordinary poultry production but can be produced experimentally. Typical symptoms of the experimentally produced disease in chickens are a decrease in appetite, a loss of weight, general paralysis and a peculiar raising and drawing back of the head. There is no evidence of an actual degeneration of the nerves such as was attributed to vitamin B_1 deficiency by earlier workers

Vitamin B_6

Little is known about the requirements of poultry for this vitamin or the symptoms of a deficiency, which infact does not occur under ordinary conditions.

Vitamin D

This vitamin is required for the normal metabolism of calcium and phosphorus in the chicken. A deficiency in the diet of growing chickens produces the abnormal condition of the bones known as rickets; in the adult chicken it causes a thinning of the egg shells and, in severe cases a decrease in egg production and hatchability. Various other conditions can cause abnormal bone development (rickets or osteoporosis), but vitamin D deficiency is the most common cause in poultry. As Titus points out, it was impossible to raise poultry in strict confinement, without access to sunshine, before the importance of vitamin D in their nutrition was discovered. Now some vitamin D is commonly included in the diet whether the birds have access to sunshine or not. The usual sources are cod-liver oil, sardine oil, certain other fish oils and D-activated animal sterol. Titus gives the amounts of the vitamin required, as well as the amounts contained in various commonly used sources.

Vitamin E

Crazy chick disease (nutritional encephalomalacia), which is usually characterized by extensive tissue changes in the brain, has been produced in chicks, ducklings and poults by feeding a diet high in fat but very low in vitamin E. It occasionally occurs in commercial flocks, perhaps through destruction or inactivation of vitamin E in feed kept too long. Titus recommends feeding mixtures while they are fresh and avoiding excessive quantities of cod-liver oil or other fats and oils in the diet. The disease can be checked in a flock and some cases can be cured, by feeding 1 percent of the oil extracted from corn, soyabeans, peanuts, wheat germ, or cottonseed. Another condition produced experimentally by Vitamin E deficiency is nutritional myopathy, a disease involving the skeletal muscles in ducklings and the muscles of the gizzard in poults.

Vitamin G

This vitamin plays a basic role in cell processes, and available evidence indicates that the growing chick requires it for the normal functioning and maintenance of the nervous system. A partial deficiency in chicks results in a condition known as curled toe paralysis as well as other symptoms, including marked adverse effects on growth; in turkey poults, a skin inflammation occurs. Since relatively few feedstuffs contain enough vitamin G to meet minimum needs during the first few weeks of life, it should be provided by careful selection of feeds. Titus gives requirements and the amounts contained in various rich sources.

Vitamin K

Apparently, vitamin K is needed for the formation of prothrombin, which in turn is necessary for the normal clotting of blood. Hemorrhages occur in very young chicks fed an experimental diet deficient in the vitamin. No deficiency is likely to occur under ordinary conditions.

Pantothenic Acid

Observations indicate that this vitamin or vitamin like factor is necessary for the maintenance of a normal spinal cord in the growing chick. A deficient diet fed experimentally produces, among other symptoms, a characteristic skin condition around the corners of the mouth and on the soles of the feet. Possibly some skin conditions seen in poultry flocks are due to a deficiency of pantothenic acid, such as might occur with certain diets. Titus gives the requirements tentatively set and the amounts in some of the rich sources. He also describes a condition called egg-white injury which closely resembles pantothenic acid deficiency but appears to be due to a deficiency of biotin (vitamin H).

Manganese and Choline

It is now known that manganese and choline (a substance found in most animal and plant tissues) somehow have a combined action in the development of a normal skeleton. Choline is seldom deficient in poultry diets; manganese, however, can easily be deficient unless the birds have access to the natural source, the soil. A deficiency of manganese (or choline, or both) in the diet of chicks, poults and ducklings produces perosis, also called hock disease and sliped tendon, characterized, among other symptoms, by enlarged joints and bending of the shank and drumstick bones. In mature birds, eggshells tend to become thin; in severe cases egg production is reduced, embryonic mortality is high and the embryos are abnormal in development. Titus gives directions for including enough manganese sulfate in the diet, mixed with salt, to serve as insurance against perosis.

Iron and Copper

Anemia rarely if ever occurs among chickens under ordinary conditions. It has been produced experimentally by feeding a diet extremely deficient in iron or copper or both, as well as by a deficiency of some unknown nutritional factor. Anemic embryos are sometimes encountered and there is evidence that lack of sunshine, or of cod-liver oil in the diet, reduces the transfer of iron and copper to the eggs.

Iodine

Goiter has been produced experimentally in chickens by feeding a diet low in iodine, and it has been reported to occur in Montana and Minnesota. It is probably more common in certain parts of the country than is generally realized. Titus suggests that the use of iodized salt for poultry may be a worth-while insurance, at least in areas where goiter occurs in either farm animals.

Gizzard Erosion

A weakening of the gizzard lining occurs commonly in chicks and is of several distinct types, apparently due to different causes. It seems to have no ill effects but probably indicates a somewhat unsatisfactory diet if it continues after the chicks are 4 weeks old. Titus lists several substances reported to be of value in clearing up the condition.

Feather Picking and Cannibalism

Cannibalism in a flock is more serious than feather picking and nearly always leads to heavy losses. Experiments indicate that diets very low in crude fiber content are a likely cause. The use of ruby lights in place of ordinary lights and the feeding of a diet containing 20 percent of barley or oats or 30 percent of bran and middlings are reported to be useful preventives. Titus gives directions for the use of salt to cure birds of these practices and for trimming back the beaks if the salt cure fails to produce results.

Fluorine and Selenium Poisoning

Fluorine poisoning depresses the rate of growth and egg production but does not occur in chickens unless the drinking water contains a certain percentage of fluorine, or unless rock phosphate or phosphatic limestone that contains fluorine is included in the diet. Selenium poisoning has several serious effects. As Titus points out, selenium has been found in the soils and vegetation in at least 11 States and probably occurs in others.

Diseases of Unknown Origin

Titus describes several conditions, encountered for the most part in experimental work, that apparently have dietary causes, not yet definitely determined–an enteritis, or inflammation of the intestines, a paralysis, an arthritis and an associated leg deformity, a dermatosis and fatty degeneration of the liver.

Titus concludes his article with a brief discussion of the influence of nutritional deficiencies on growth and reproduction.

Chapter 1

PULLORUM DISEASE

Hubert Bunyea[1]

[1] *Hubert Bunyea is Veterinarian, Pathological Division, Bureau of Animal Industry.*

Here is the story of one of the most insidious and devastating of all poultry diseases and how it is being successfully combated by a determined drive on a national scale.

During the early days of the present century a new poultry disease was causing much confusion. First called a fatal chick septicemia and later bacillary white diarrhea, it is now known as pullorum disease. Among the causes to which it was attributed were chilling, overheating, poor care, coccidiosis and bacteria of indefinite types. The incubator also came in for a share of the blame. The origin of the disease was shrouded in mystery, probably because it was masked by the multitude of conditions with which it was confused. The first step toward its control came in 1900 and 1901 when Rettger[2] announced the discovery of the causative organism, *Salmonella pullorum*. Since Rettger's memorable contribution, pullorum disease has been made the subject of an enormous amount of scientific research, as attested by the 400 to 500 references to it in technical literature.

---

[2] RETTGER, LEO F. SEPTICEMIA AMONG YOUNG CHICKENS and SEPTICEMIA IN YOUNG CHICKENS. N.Y. Med, Jour. 71: 803-805, illus., and 73: 267-268, illus. 1900 and 1901.

Economic Importance

The disease is important from an economic standpoint because it injures the productivity of hens and lowers the livability of chicks. From the medical standpoint as well as the economic, it is important, because the infection in the ovary, to which pullorum disease is usually confined in hens, is transmitted to some of the eggs and to the chicks hatched from these eggs. The resulting mortality among chicks is at time enormous. The damage is increased by the fact that chicks from healthy hens may also acquire the disease by contact with infected chicks in incubators and brooders, as well as under hens. Infected chicks are constantly voiding enormous numbers of the germs in their droppings, thereby spreading the infection.

The chicks from infected eggs may die in the shell or a short time after hatching. Some diseased chicks may survive for only 2 or 3 weeks, whereas others live to maturity and perpetuate the disease by harbouring the germ in their egg organs and infecting their eggs and chicks.

Although definite statistics on the annual losses to the poultry industry in the United States from pullorum disease are not available, it is known that the disease exists in every part of the country and probably in every locality where appreciable numbers of poultry are kept. It would be impossible to estimate the cost of the disease to the industry through the death of baby chicks alone, not to mention diminished egg production in hens and pullets, reduced hatchability of eggs and occasionally the death of hens due to generalized pullorum infection.

Cause, Occurrence and Symptoms

The disease is caused by the toxin-forming germ *Salmonella pullorum*. Although this germ is easily destroyed, it has been known to remain alive in soil or manure in sheltered places for many days, or even for months. The primary seat of infection is the ovary of the infected hen. Although the disease is commonly transmitted from the hen to the chick by means of the egg, not every egg laid by an infected, or carrier, hen contains the germ. Infected eggs, if hatched, are likely to produce infected chicks.

Besides occurring in chickens, pullorum disease within recent years has come to have increased importance as an infection of turkeys. It has also been observed in a few instances in ducks, sparrows, European bullfinches, pigeons, quail, geese, pheasants, bittern, peafowl, goldfinches, greenfinches, green canaries; turtledoves, guinea fowl and rabbits. Human beings and other mammals are not known to be affected.

In hens and pullets, pullorum disease is as a rule localized in the egg-making organs and produces no outward symptoms. It may, therefore, exist unsuspected in a breeder flock. In chicks the symptoms of the disease and the deaths it causes are sometimes wrongly attributed to some other cause, such as fungus pneumonia (as per gillosis), ceiling and overheating. The description of its principal characteristics which follows furnishes some means of recognizing the presence of the disease. It is not to be assumed, however, that a definite diagnosis can be made by the symptoms alone. In order to diagnose the disease beyond question, clinical observations must be confirmed in most cases by bacteriological proof.

Pullorum disease is observed in chicks from the time of hatching until they are about 3 weeks old or older. The chicks may die suddenly after showing slight symptoms for a short time. Generally, however, they first seem disposed to huddle together or to remain too much of the time under the hen or the hover. They soon appear drowsy and indifferent to their surroundings. They stand with closed eyes and ruffled plumage, list lessly picking at their feed from time to time but apparently not eating it (Fig. 1). Their droppings may be whitish, foamy and sticky but are sometimes brownish in colour; the name "bacillary white diarrhea" is in some cases an inaccurate description. Sometimes the excreta stick to the down around the vent and accumulate until they completely cover and plug the opening (Fig. 2). This condition, known as "pasting up behind," unless soon relieved, will quickly cause the death of chicks. When attempting to void excrement, the sick chicks utter shrill cries of pain. Laboured abdominal breathing signals the approach of death, which may come quickly or after a period of extreme prostration. The death rate in infected broods may range from 50 to 80 percent or even higher.

In baby chicks infected in the egg, symptoms and death may occur immediately after hatching or in a day or so. Chicks that contract the disease after hatching show symptoms in 6 to 8 days, or even later. Deaths may occur from the time of hatching until about 3 weeks later, when the brood may be practically exterminated.

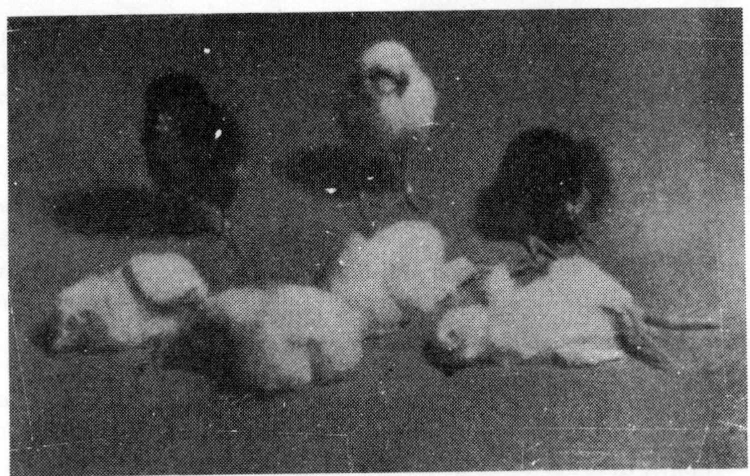

Fig. 1: Chicks sick and dead from pullorum disease. The sick ones show such symptoms as drowsiness, depression, and drooping wings.

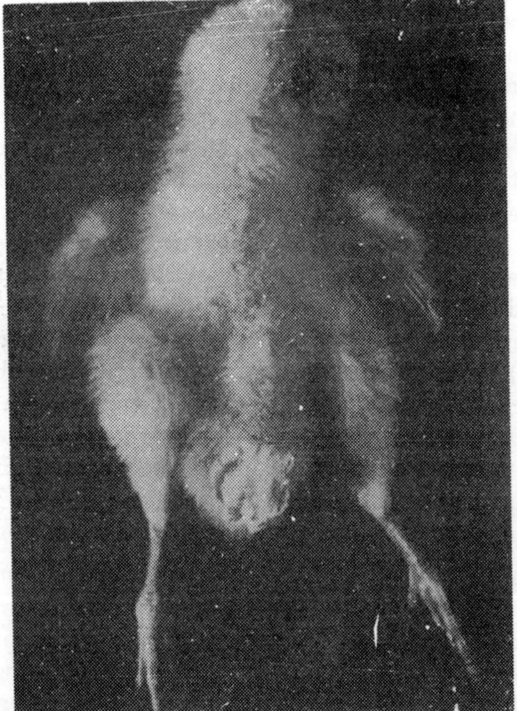

Fig. 2: Chick dead from pullorum disease, showing occlusion of vent with mucilaginons excreta characteristic of this disease.

Not all pullorum-infected chicks die young; if this were the case, the disease would be self-limiting. Unfortunately, many infected chicks survive to maturity and harbour the infection in their eggmaking organs and as a result many of their chicks die and the disease is perpetuated in at least some of those that survive. Some pullorum-infected embryos die in the shell.

Post Mortem Findings

In hens and pullets the outstanding change brought about by the disease is that seen in the ovary on post mortem examination or when the carcass is dressed. In an advanced case of pullorum infection, the partly or wholly developed yolks are angular in outline (Fig. 3), shrunken, hard and of an abnormal brownish or greenish colour. Yolks containing dark fluid are sometimes seen. The presence of the germ in diseased *ova* can be demonstrated readily by labouratory methods. In incipient cases, the infection may exist in ovaries of apparently normal appearance.

In a chick dead from pullorum disease, the presence of noticeable changes depends somewhat on the age of the chick. Chicks 1 to 5 days old often fail to show visible internal evidences of the disease. Chicks dying at 6 days of age and upwards often have small spots of destroyed tissue, like whitish deposits, in the lungs, in the muscles of the heart and occasionally on the outer surface of the intestines.

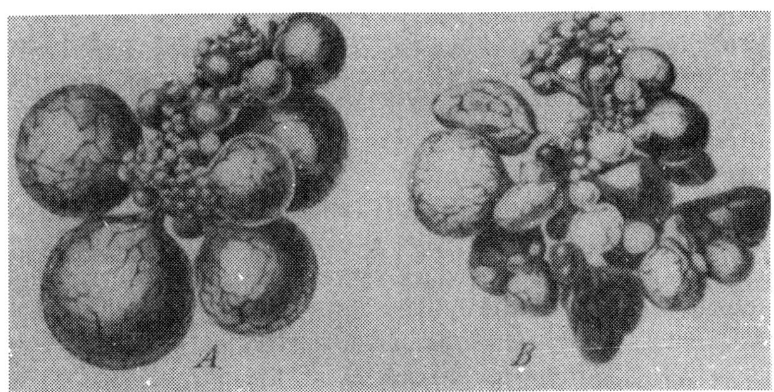

Fig. 3: *A*: Normal ovary of fowl; *B*: ovary affected with *Salmonella pullorum* (After Rettger).

Early writers ascribed importance to pneumonia, ocher-coloured livers and unabsorbed yolks as evidences of the disease in chicks, but later research has shown that these symptoms occur irrespective of pullorum infection. On the other hand, the absence of an pathological changes observable on autopsy does not exclude the possibility that the disease is present. Only by bacteriological examination of the dead chick can the presence or absence of pullorum infection be definitely determined. The germs sometimes in habit practically every organ in the chick's body, but they are most frequently sought for and recovered from the heart blood, liver, lungs and unabsorbed portions of yolk.

The technique of demonstrating the presence of this infection in fowls of any age requires highly specialized training, as well as the use of equipment and materials not generally available outside a labouratory. It is usually possible to obtain an expert bacteriological examination of suspected cases of pullorum disease at any of the various State agricultural experiment stations.

Dissemination in Incubators or Brooders

Pullorum disease has existed for many years in the United States, but its economic importance increased with the recent tremendous development of the hatching industry. Medical science has shown that pullorum disease is capable of spreading from infected to healthy chicks in all the various types of incubators in common use when some of the eggs hatched are from infected parent stock. The shells of infected eggs and the fluff or down which the newly hatched chicks shed may also contain the infection; hence, it often happens that the hatching of pullorum-infected eggs in an incubator results in widespread transmission of the disease to other chicks hatched from uninfected eggs in the same incubator. Infected chicks will also spread the disease to healthy chicks in a brooder house. Pullorum-infected eggs will produce diseased chicks under a hen just as in an incubator and the disease may also spread to the healthy chicks of the brood. In the hatchery chick, however, the danger of acquiring the disease is multiplied by the fact that the eggs for hatching are frequently assembled from a number of flocks and if one or more of these flocks harbour the disease agent, the entire output of the incubator is exposed to infection.

Through the hatchery, from which chicks are distributed over a wide territory, the disease may be disseminated over large areas and may cause enormous losses to the poultry industry. The hatcheryman therefore has a responsibility, which he has not been slow to recognize and concerning which there is much that he can do, both to conserve the stability of his own enterprise and to serve the best interests of the poultrymen on whom his success depends. Many progressive hatcherymen have already realized the importance of taking the initiative in controlling pullorum disease in their communities by requiring the flocks that supply them with eggs to be tested for the presence of pullorum disease carriers.

Transmission Among Adults

It is well known that resistance to pullorum infection increases with the age of the chick and that many adult fowls remain healthy among infected ones. Occasional instances of transmission of the disease among adult fowls occur, however, particularly if the birds are crowded or the infection is concentrated.

Proof that pullorum disease is transmissible from infected hens to normal hens or pullets was obtained in an experiment conducted by the United States Department of Agriculture. Twelve pullets free from pullorum disease were allowed to mingle for 7 months with 35 hens which were shown to be infected with the disease by their reaction to the agglutination test, described later. The two groups were then separated and mated to non-reactor cockerels. During the following 2 months the hens were trap-nested and their eggs were saved for hatching. Bacteriological examinations of the dead embryos, the baby chicks that died within 2 weeks after hatching and the exposed pullets showed that half the exposed pullets acquired the disease from the infected hens. Similar examination confirmed the presence of the disease in the 35 originally infected hens. Such evidence shows that under conditions of concentrated infection, pullorum disease is transmissible from infected to normal hens irrespective of the influence of the male birds.

Control Measures

Since the invention of the mammoth incubator in recent years, poultry production has advanced to a high position in agriculture and the hatchery industry has assumed gigantic proportions. This development has intensified the problem of pullorum disease control, one of the most serious confronting the hatchery industry. It is obvious, however, that the control of pullorum disease is not primarily an incubator problem but one of flock hygiene and that its solution in the main depends not on special appliances or procedures in the hatching of eggs or the brooding of chicks but rather on the successful diagnosis of the disease in carrier adults, so that such adults may be eliminated or excluded from breeding flocks.

No known medicinal treatment or method of vaccination is of value in the prevention or cure of pullorum disease in chicks or hens. Indeed, the very nature of the disease renders treatment both futile and undesirable. Flocks harbouring the infection should not be used for breeding purposes. The fact that the cycle of infection (Fig. 4) includes the diseased hen, the infected egg, the surviving infected baby chick and the diseased pullet indicates that it is not advisable to save for breeders any chicks that have recovered from an attack of pullorum disease. Hens that harbour the infection in their ovaries are likely to lay infected eggs from which diseased

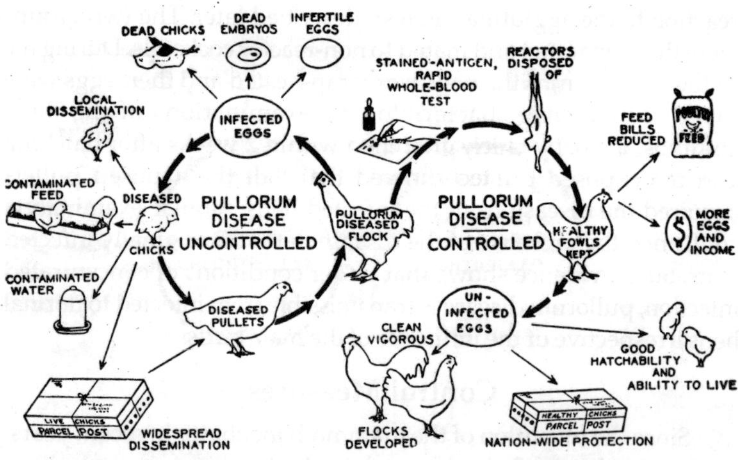

Fig. 4: Comparison of injurious effects of un-controlled pullorum disease with benefits resulting from the application of the agglutination test and the disposal of reactors.

chicks will be hatched. The only practicable means of controlling pullorum disease, therefore, is to detect the carrier hens and eliminate them from the breeding flock.

Diagnosis

The clinical diagnosis of the carrier state in pullorum control is made difficult by reason of the fact, already noted that the infection is usually localized in the ovary of the hen or pullet and betrays no outward evidence of its presence. In fact, the pullorum infected hen is frequently one of the healthiest looking birds in the flock.

Two methods of detecting pullorum disease carriers have been developed, namely, the agglutination test and the intradermic, or wattle, test. Since its adaptation to diagnosis of this disease in 1913, the agglutination test has been almost universally accepted as the most satisfactory method available for the diagnosis of the infection in fowls of breeding age. Repeated comparative experimental tests have demonstrated its superiority to the intradermic test. Like most other diagnostic tests, however, it is admittedly not infallible. It has been employed in various parts of the country with such variations in technique and interpretation as to make errors inevitable in some instances. Improvement in this respect has gradually followed the standardization of test methods; and uniformity of equipment, technique and interpretation of results is little by little being achieved in the various testing labouratories.

The tests must be carried out by technically trained persons, but because many poultry producers and hatcherymen are interested in knowing about the techniques used, the following descriptions given.

The Agglutination Test

Three different forms of agglutination test are in use at present:

(1) The long method, or tube test,

(2) The rapid serum test, and

(3) The stained-antigen, rapid whole-blood test.

For practical purposes the three may be considered about equally reliable for the detection of pullorum disease.

The Long Method, or Tube Test

This test for pullorum disease has been in use since 1913, when it was developed by Jones.[3] It is at present officially recognized and used in several of the States engaged in combating the disease. For this test, clear serum is obtained from each fowl to be tested and the samples are so packed as to avoid spoilage and breakage during shipment to the labouratory.

In the labouratory the serum is distributed in one or more test tubes in measured amounts. In each test tube is then placed another fluid called the antigen, which has previously been prepared from cultures of selected strains of *Salmonella pullorum*.

Measured amounts of the antigen are added to measured amounts of the diluted serum in test tubes and incubated at 37°C. Readings are then made and recorded. Tubes showing doubtful or suspicious reactions are held at room temperature for an additional 24 hours, after which the final reading is made.

Positive agglutination (Fig. 5, *A*) involves the complete clearing of the fluid and the clumping of the hitherto suspended matter in the bottom of the tube. A doubtful reaction (Fig. 5, *B*) should always be reported as suspicious and the fowl should be retested or removed from the flock. Results are negative (Fig. 5, *C*) when there is no clearing and no separation of the suspended matter.

Some diagnostic labouratories modify this procedure in various ways. The test has been found to be rather expensive and in many of the States no facilities are available for its application. The tube test was adopted in 1932 by the United States Live Stock Sanitary Association as a standard method.[4]

---

[3] JONES, F.S. THE VALUE OF THE MACROSCOPIC AGGLUTINATION TEST IN DETECTING FOWLS THAT ARE HARBORING BACTERIUM PULLORUM. N.Y. State Vet. Col. Rept. 1911-12, pp. 149-158. 1913. See also Jour. Med. Res. 27: 481-495. 1913.

[4] The standard tube agglutination test. REPORT OF THE CONFERENCE OF OFFICIAL RESEARCH WORKERS IN ANIMAL DISEASES. II. SEROLOGICAL DIAGNOSIS OF PULLORUM DISEASE (CARRIER CONDITION) IN MATURING AND IN ADULT BREEDING STOCK. Amer. Vet. Med. Assoc. Jour. 82: 488-490. 1933.

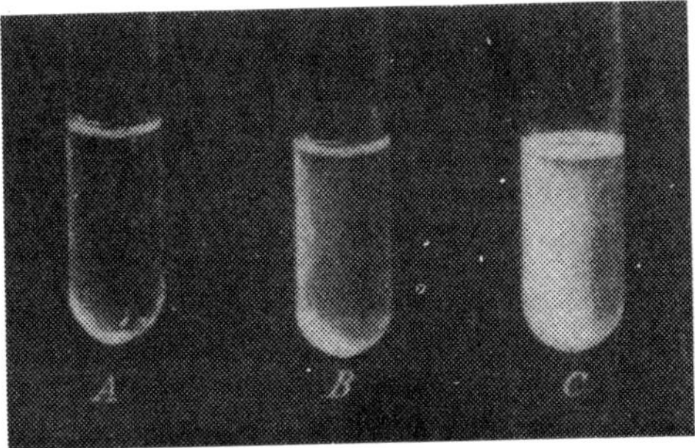

Fig. 5: Tube agglutination test reactions for pullorum disease. *A*: positive reaction; *B*: suspicious or doubtful reaction, *C*: negative reaction.

With a view to reducing the cost of poultry testing to the flock owner and thus placing the test within the reach of a larger part of the industry, research workers have within recent years developed rapid agglutination-test methods.

The Rapid Serum Test

This method of testing fowls for pullorum disease was originally described by Runnells and his associates[5] in 1927. The undiluted clear serum of the fowl to be tested is mixed with a highly concentrated antigen on a pane of glass ruled in 1 inch squares which forms the top of a box, black on the inside and illuminated by a frosted incandescent bulb within. Two squares on the glass are used for each sample of clear serum to be tested. Amounts of the serum used are 0.02 cubic centimeter and 0.01 cubic centimeter, respectively and 0.02 cubic centimeter of antigen is used in each case. The two substances are mixed with a toothpick. The reaction may occur immediately or may require several minutes. A positive reaction consists in the formation of visible clumps of the bacteria suspended in the antigen and a clearing of the intervening fluid. A

---

[5] RUNNELLS, R.A., COON, C.J., FARLEY, H., and THORP, F. AN APPLICATION OF THE RAPID-METHOD AGGLUTINATION TEST TO THE DIAGNOSIS OF BACILLARY WHITE DIARRHEA INFECTION. Amer, Vet. Med. Assoc. Jour. 70: 660-662. 1927.

negative test remains uniformly cloudy without the formation of clumps. Because it requires clear serum for testing, this method is essentially a labouratory procedure, but under certain circumstances it may be made adaptable to field use.

The Stained-antigen, Rapid Whole-blood Test

This test, which was developed by workers in the Bureau of Animal Industry[6], is somewhat similar in its technique to the rapid serum test. Outstanding features of the rapid whole-blood test are the following:

(1) The use of a single drop of fresh whole blood immediately after it is obtained from the fowl.

(2) The use of a stained antigen, which makes reacting samples easily detectable over a white background without artificial illumination.

(3) The fact that the presence or absence of pullorum infection is immediately diagnosed in one handling of the fowl and reactors are disposed of at the time of the test, which eliminates the necessity of re-handling or banding the fowls.

The antigen for the rapid whole-blood test is stained with an aqueous solution of crystal violet.

In applying this test a drop of blood is secured by pricking the wing vein with a sharp-pointed instrument or in any other convenient manner. The drop of blood is picked up by the aid of a loop of fine wire. A drop of stained antigen is placed on a white glass plate. A loopful of blood is taken up from the wing vein. The blood is then stirred into the antigen and the mixture spread to a diameter of about 1 inch. The loop is then rinsed in clean water and dried by touching it to a piece of clean blotting paper if necessary.

The glass plate is rocked from side to side a few times to mix the antigen and blood thoroughly and to facilitate agglutination. The reaction is usually visible in 5 seconds to 2 minutes. Slight reactions which require more than 2 minutes should be disregarded.

---

6 SCHAFFER, J.M., MacDONALD, A.D. HALL, W.J., and BUNYEA, H. A STAINED ANTIGEN FOR THE RAPID WHOLE BLOOD TEST FOR PULLORUM DISEASE. Amer. Vet. Med. Assoc. Jour., 79; 236-240. 1931.

Various degrees of reaction are observed in this as in other agglutination tests (Fig. 6). The greater the agglutinating power of the blood, the more rapid the clumping and the larger the clumps. A positive reaction (Fig 6, *A*) consists in a clumping of the antigen in well-developed flocculi (separated particles) surrounded by clear spaces. This reaction is easily distinguished against a white background. A somewhat weaker reaction (Fig. 6, *B*) consists of small but still clearly visible clumps of antigen surrounded by spaces only partly clear. The interpretation of these partial or suspicious reactions should be the same as that of similarly incomplete tube-method agglutination reactions. Between this point and a negative reaction (Fig. 6, *D*) there sometimes occurs a very fine granulation barely visible to the naked eye (Fig. 6, *C*); this should be disregarded in making a diagnosis. In a non-reactor the smear remains homogeneous. The very fine, marginal flocculation (separation of particles) which may occur just before the sample dries up is also regarded as negative.

A white glass plate has proved most satisfactory for this work. The use of the plate enables the tester to have a number of successive test mixtures under observation without delaying the work to wait for results before proceeding to the next bird. As a result of long experience in testing with this antigen. It has been decided to regard as definitely positive only those reactions that appear within 1

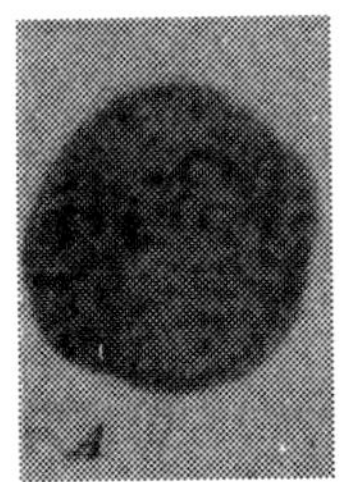

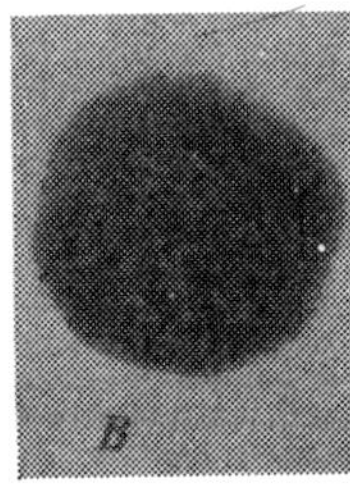

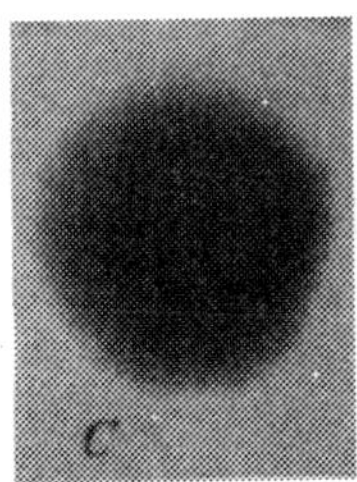

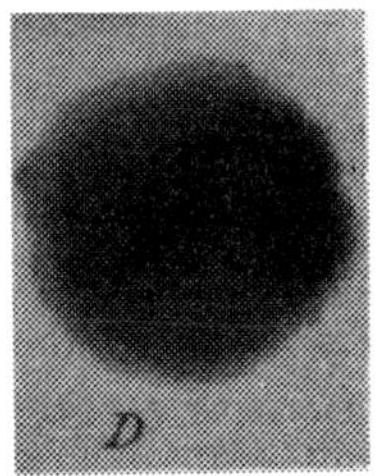

Fig. 6: Reactions to the stained-antigen, rapid whole-blood test. *A*: a positive reaction; *B*: a doubtful or suspicious reaction; *C*: a false. or pin-point reaction; *D*: a negative reaction.

minute after mixing the antigen and blood, while those appearing within 2 minutes are regarded as suspicious.

The Intradermic Test

This method, which was described by Ward and Gallagher[7] in 1917, consists in injecting into the dermis, or skin of the wattle a small amount of a diagnostic agent prepared from a broth culture of *Salmonella pullorum*. The product is prepared by incubating a broth culture of *S. pullorum* for about a month, after which it is preserved by the addition of 0.5 percent of phenol and held for several weeks before use.

In applying the test, the fluid is injected slightly above the lower border of the wattle. In reacting cases an edematous, or watery swelling of the injected wattle appears after approximately 24 hours. Although the results reported by Ward and Gallagher were in some measure discordant with the results of the agglutination test and the autopsy findings, these authors believed that the intradermic test had showed sufficient promise to warrant further extensive trial in the field in comparison with the agglutination test.

A number of investigators have at different times pursued more advanced comparative researches with this method of testing fowls for pullorum disease. None, however, have thus far been successful in developing the test to a degree of accuracy comparable to that of the agglutination-test methods.

Pullorum Disease in Turkeys

The problem of controlling pullorum disease in turkeys has several aspects that make it different from the control problem in chickens.

The first is the behavior of the disease in turkeys. The scientific evidence now available indicates that turkey poults are very susceptible and suffer a high mortality when exposed to the disease. Such outbreaks in poults have in many instances been attributed to the fact that they were hatched in the same incubator or brooded in the same quarters with pullorum-diseased chicks. Other outbreaks

---

[7] WARD, A.R., and GALLAGHER, B.A. AN INTRADERMAL TEST FOR BACTERIUM PULLORUM INFECTION IN FOWLS. U.S. Dept. Agr. Dept. Bull. 517, 15 pp. 1917.

have been traced directly to pullorum infection harboured in the ovaries of breeding turkey hens.

The adult turkey may not ordinarily be a natural host for *Salmonella pullorum*. The germ has been found, however, at autopsy in turkeys that reacted to the agglutination test for pullorum disease, as well as in eggs from reacting turkeys. In a number of outbreaks of pullorum disease in turkey poults it has been found that the condition was not transmitted through the eggs from infected dams. Adult turkeys that have reacted to the test tend to become either partly or completely negative to it within a year or less, suggesting that the turkey is an unfavorable host for the infection and is therefore able to overcome it as the chicken cannot.

The stained-antigen, rapid whole-blood test was developed for the testing of chickens for pullorum disease, but within recent years the method has been used to some extent in testing adult turkeys also for this disease. The stained antigen for chickens has not been found altogether satisfactory for turkeys, however and experiments are under way in the Bureau of Animal Industry looking to the development of a suitable stained antigen for testing turkeys. At present, the tube-agglutination test is probably the most satisfactory method.

The operation of a general blood-testing programme for pullorum disease control in turkeys is beset with complicating considerations. Other germs, of both disease-producing and harmless species, are able to cause the turkey's blood to react to the pullorum disease agglutination test. The injection of certain bacterins (vaccines prepared from bacteria) may cause the bird to give a false pullorum disease reaction for as long as 1 or 2 months; hence, the pullorum, disease test is very difficult to interpret in turkeys. Where evidence exists that an occasional breeding flock has become accidentally infected, however, some investigators advise that the flock be tested and the reactors removed before eggs are saved for hatching. Such incidents may largely be averted by hatching turkey eggs separately from chicken eggs in properly disinfected incubators and by brooding poults entirely apart from chicks. It seems advisable from the standpoint of a Nation-wide programme of control of pullorum disease in turkeys to place the emphasis on the importance of separate hatching and separate brooding.

Pullorum Control Under the National Poultry Improvement Plan

The losses from pullorum disease were so great that the need for organized efforts to control it was early recognized. By 1925 a number of the States had inaugurated programmes to that end. Although much good was accomplished, it soon became apparent that the diversity of terminology and of methods would eventually lead to chaos. Leaders in the movement began to think about a properly co-ordinated, nationally sponsored programme in which the terminology would be uniform and the objectives and procedures could be intelligently guided into definite, constructive and mutually advantageous channels.

Numerous State, regional and national conferences were held by members of the industry at key points and as a result the National Poultry Improvement Plan was inaugurated July 1, 1935. The plan is administered by official State agencies in each of the voluntarily participating States in co-operation with the Bureau of Animal Industry. The aim is in part to establish a workable pullorum-control programme in each State. Each State agency is responsible not only for carrying out the breeding stages of the plan but also for the systematic testing of participating flocks for pullorum disease.

Although the application of the pullorum control and eradication phase of the plan has heretofore been optional with the individual States, beginning September 1, 1943, all flocks in the plan must be officially tested for pullorum disease.

The three agglutination-test methods described are given equal recognition in the pullorum-control plan. All pullorum testing under the plan is performed by individuals properly trained and authorized by the official State agency.

The testing is done by a livestock sanitary authority, an official of the State college of agriculture, or a similarly authorized State employee. In the U.S. Pullorum-Tested and U.S. Pullorum-Controlled classes, special provisions enable the work to be done by a pullorum-testing agent who has been officially trained and authorized to do this work.

There are four pullorum-control and eradication classes: U.S. Pullorum-Tested, U.S. Pullorum-Controlled, U.S. Pullorum-Passed and U.S. Pullorum-Clean. Tolerance of pullorum reactors in the U.S. Pullorum-Tested class in the 1941-42 testing year is required to be less than 9 percent and this percentage is to decrease 1 percent a year until it is less than 5 percent, which will occur in the fall of 1945. Reactors must have been removed from the premises before hatching eggs may be saved. All birds over 5 months of age to be used as breeders must be tested.

In the U.S. Pullorum-Controlled class the number of reactors tolerated in the last test must be fewer than 2 percent of the flock. The test must be made within 12 months immediately preceding the date of sale of hatching eggs or chicks from such flock. All chickens over 5 months of age to be used as breeders must be tested.

In the U.S. Pullorum-Passed and the U.S. Pullorum-Clean classes, no reactors may be found in any test. In the U.S. Pullorum-Passed class, all birds 5 months of age or older must be tested within the testing year immediately preceding the date of sale of hatching eggs or chicks. In the U.S. Pullorum-Clean class, no reactors may be found in either of two consecutive tests not less than 6 months apart, the last test being made within the testing year immediately preceding the date of sale of hatching eggs or chicks. In this class all chickens over 5 months of age to be used as breeders must be tested.

The participation of the States in the various pullorum-control classes has increased each year since the inauguration of the plan, beginning with 30 States in 1935-36 and reaching a total of 44 in 1940-41. The number of birds officially tested in accordance with the provisions of the plan increased from 2,058,782 during the first year to 10,527,946 birds during the sixth year, 1940-41. During the year ended June 30, 1941, approximately three-fourths of the birds were in the U.S. Pullorum-Tested class.

Although definite chick-mortality statistics are not available, reports from the industry all over the country indicate that the hatchability of eggs is gradually improving and mortality among chicks is steadily decreasing as a result of the pullorum-control phase of the National Poultry Improvement Plan.

An individual poultryman, or hatcheryman who desires to have the benefit of the pullorum test for his breeding flock or flocks may do one of several things:

(1) He may become a participant in the National Poultry Improvement Plan by complying with the preliminary requirements in his State. The application for participation should be made to the official State agency of the National Poultry Improvement Plan, whose exact name and post-office address may be obtained from county agricultural agents, State agricultural extension services, State departments of agriculture, or the Bureau of Animal Industry at Washington, D.C.

(2) Individuals who do not care to participate in the National Poultry Improvement Plan may have their flocks tested privately by applying to their State veterinarian or to the agricultural experiment station, which is affiliated with their State agricultural college. In many States, practicing veterinarians may be called upon for such service.

It is not advisable for persons not properly trained in the use of pullorum antigen to undertake to perform the test on their own hens or those of other persons.

Chapter 2

FOWL PARALYSIS AND OTHER FORMS OF THE AVIAN LEUKOSIS COMPLEX

C.A. Brandly, Nelson F. Water & W.J. Hall[1]

[1] *C.A. Brandly is Senior Pathologist and Nelson F. Waters is Senior Geneticist, Regional Poultry Research Labouratory, East Lansing, Mich. and W.J. Hall is Veterinarian, Beltsville Research Center, Beltsville, Md., Bureau of Animal Industry.*

Fowl Paralysis is one form of a very damaging disease complex that probably costs poultrymen in the United States as much as all other diseases put together. No one knows what causes it, how it spreads, or how to control it. This article tells about a concerted drive to discover more facts, with a view to reducing a tremendous annual loss.

The disease called fowl paralysis, together with several other allied conditions classed together as the avian leukosis complex,[2] causes a tremendous loss to the poultry industry. The paralysis form

---

[2] In the avian leukosis complex may be included in addition to so-called fowl paralysis, or range paralysis, also termed neurolymphomatosis, other forms of lymphomatosis; ocular lymphomatosis, or iritis; visceral lymphomatosis, or big-liver disease; lymphocytoma, myelocytoma, and leukotic tumors; osteopetrosis, or marble bone; and the leukoses-erythroleukosis, erythrosis, myeloleukosis,

of this disease complex was first recognized in the United States along the eastern coast about 1920.

During the last 20 years the avian leukosis complex has spread rapidly until few flocks of chickens in the United States have escaped its ravages. Its yearly toll in this country is believed to exceed that of any other poultry disease and it also causes great damage in other countries of the world where the production of poultry is conducted on a considerable scale. Although chickens from a few weeks old to a year of age or older may become affected, the disease usually does not appear to a great extent in flocks until after the expense of rearing has been incurred. It is partly for this reason that the disease exacts such a great financial toll. The control of the avian leukosis complex consequently is of major interest to all concerned with the poultry industry.

With the aim of finding some means to reduce losses from this disease, investigations are being actively carried out by various State and Federal workers.

Types and Symptoms

One of the most obvious symptoms of the avian leukosis complex is a paralyzed condition in one or more parts of a bird's body. This led early workers to call the disease fowl paralysis. Later examinations and study revealed a great variety of apparently closely related disease manifestations. Practically all the tissues, organs and other parts of the body have been found to be involved. The numerous expressions of disease make it desirable to use the more inclusive term "avian-leukosis complex," of which paralysis, or nerve involvement, is only one type or manifestation.

The various types of the leukosis complex may be classified as (1) nerve (neural), (2) eye (ocular); (3) internal-organ (visceral), (4) bone and (5) blood (leukosis). It should be emphasized that a

---

Footnote Contd.

erythromyeloblastic or erythroblastic, and granuloblastic leukosis, etc. These diseases or expressions of disease show differences in various features; yet marked similarities exist among certain of their characteristics. These resemblances are taken as a basis for a common group or name, although the knowledge of the relation- ship which one type or form of disease may have to another within the complex is quite limited.

bird may be affected by one or all these types at the same time. In addition, other unrelated diseases may also be present. These facts greatly complicate the already difficult task of determining the true nature of the disease or diseases present.

The various types described in the following paragraphs may be found in both males and females and some may exist in a bird for long periods without producing any noticeable effect.

Nerve Type (Neural Lymphomatosis)

The nerve type of the disease is most familiar to the poultryman. Figure 1 shows a typical position of the legs (spraddling), which is considered characteristic. One or both legs or wings may be affected, with a resulting partial or complete paralysis of these parts. Examination of the nerves of the diseased part with the unaided eye may show great enlargement and a slight yellowish discolouration, but often the use of a microscope is necessary to detect the disease changes. The nerves of other parts of the body may also be affected, resulting in so-called sour crop, wry neck and a general in co-ordination of the entire body. Partial or complete paralysis of the viscera occurs in many cases. Breathing through the mouth or difficult respiration may be observed when the vagus nerve, which serves the lungs and stomach, is involved. The length of time an affected bird may survive depends on the extent, location and function of the nerve or nerves affected. Partially paralyzed birds have been known to live many months in individual pens with access to feed and water.

Other diseases of the fowl that produce similar or identical symptoms of paralysis may be confused with the nerve type of the avian leukosis complex. Among these are certain of the nutritional diseases, including several vitamin deficiencies and infectious diseases, such as epidemic tremor, or avian encephalomyelitis. The fact that several other diseases may show all the gross symptoms and changes of the nerve type of the avian leukosis complex indicates the need for careful diagnosis and makes it evident that the term "fowl paralysis" refers to a symptom of disease and not a disease. A final differentiation between so-called fowl paralysis, or neurolymphomatosis and paralysis resulting from other causes often requires microscopic and various additional labouratory examinations and procedures.

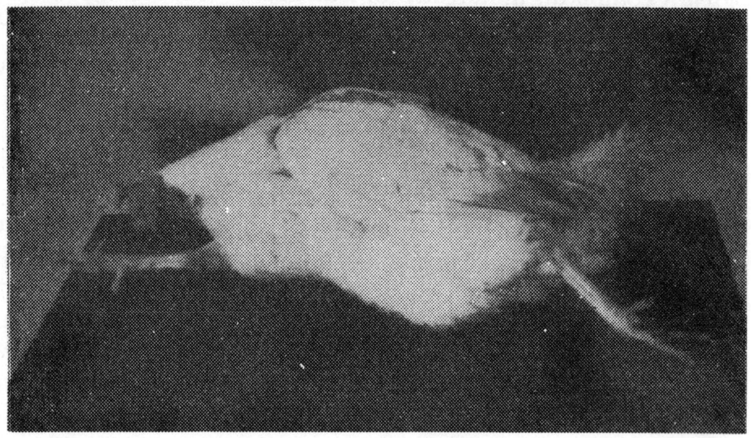

Fig. 1: Typical spraddling position of the legs in neurolymphomatosis, the nerve form of fowl paralysis.

Eye Type (Ocular Lymphomatosis)

The eye type is quite common and is frequently manifested in the bird by loss of colour in the iris and development of grey eyes and "fishy," or bulging, eyeballs (Fig. 2). Changes in the size and shape of the pupil are also commonly seen in ocular lymphomatosis. In some cases the nerves leading to the eyes are affected, with partial or complete blindness as the usual result. There is a considerable amount of variability in the time when eye disorders are manifested. They may first be observed as early as the fourth month of age, but the majority of cases occur between the fourth and twelfth months. New cases may appear, however, even after the birds are a year or more old. It should be remembered that though the iris of the eye of the adult fowl is normally pigmented, during the first few months after hatching the eye is gray or un-pigmented. Thus the lack of pigment during the early period should not be confused with loss of pigment resulting from the eye type of the leukosis complex. Since the eye changes usually develop slowly, an affected hen may remain in production until almost complete blindness interferes with its obtaining feed and water.

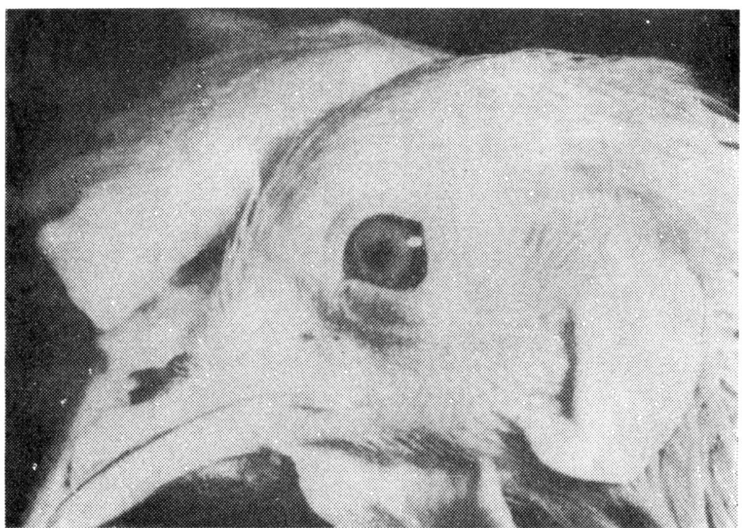

Fig. 2: Gray coloration of the iris and distortion of the pupil, called pearly eye and iritis, seen in ocular lymphomatosis, the eye type of fowl paralysis.

Internal-Organ or Visceral Type (Visceral Lymphomatosis)

Labouratory examinations indicate that all the internal organs of the bird are affected by the avian leukosis complex. The liver, lungs, heart, spleen, ovary, testicles, kidneys, intestines, skin and in fact every tissue or organ may show disease manifestations that are part of this complex (Fig. 3). All of these organs may not, however, be affected at the same time. The disease may be seen in birds from a few weeks to several years of age.

On examination the various internal organs of diseased birds frequently show gross tumorlike masses, though in some cases these "tumors" may be seen only with the aid of a microscope. An infiltration of young or immature blood cells into the liver may cause a general enlargement of this organ without a nodular, or spotted, effect. The liver may increase to several times its normal size. Livers weighing more than a pound have been found in affected birds weighing less than 4 pounds. This condition is frequently called

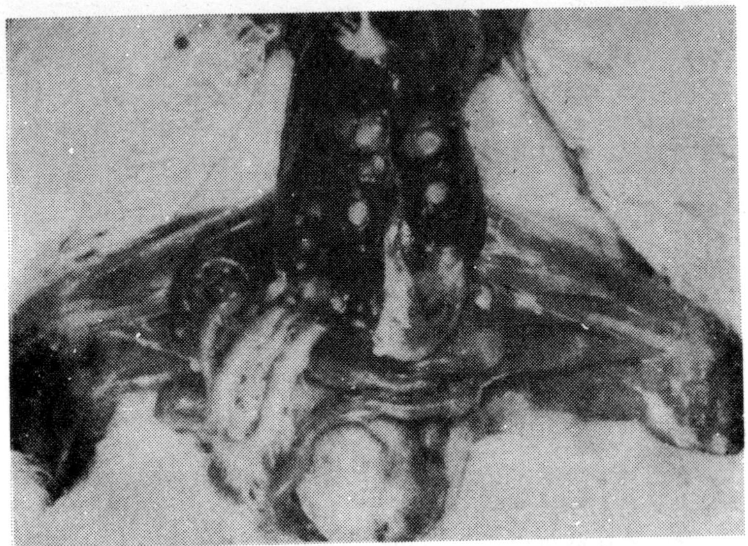

Fig. 3: Lymphoid tumors in the liver and intestines of a chicken, a result of visceral lymphomatosis.

big-liver disease. The external symptoms shown by a bird vary according to the location and extent of the disease condition. For example, when the liver is seriously affected the blood circulation and digestive system do not function normally and the bird generally lose flesh, becoming weak and non-productive. As in other forms of the leukosis complex and in other diseases, a diarrhoea often develops either as a direct consequence or as a result of complications. Death may occur either before serious external symptoms are observed or after a long period of sickness.

Various unrelated diseases may cause symptoms identical with those shown by birds affected by the visceral type of the leukosis complex. The lesions, or tissue injuries, of tuberculosis may be so similar that frequently differentiation can be made only by labouratory examinations. The fact that other forms of the leukosis complex, the nerve type, for example, may be seen in a flock suggests but does not prove that the organ, or visceral, type is present also.

Bone Type (Osteopetrosis)

A bone condition (25, 27)[3] in which the long bones (leg and wing) are thickened and enlarged without any increase in length taking place has been found to be associated with, the avian leukosis complex (Fig. 4). The walls of the bone become thickened and very hard and the amount of space normally occupied by the bone marrow is greatly diminished. In advanced cases the bone deformity of the shanks is readily noticed and affected birds have a stilted or jerky gait. The scientific name of this bone condition is osteopetrosis (literally, hardening of the bone).

Blood Types (Leukosis)

In one type of the avian leukosis complex the blood and blood-forming organs and tissues, especially the bone marrow (where blood cells are made), are affected. The blood is the direct means for

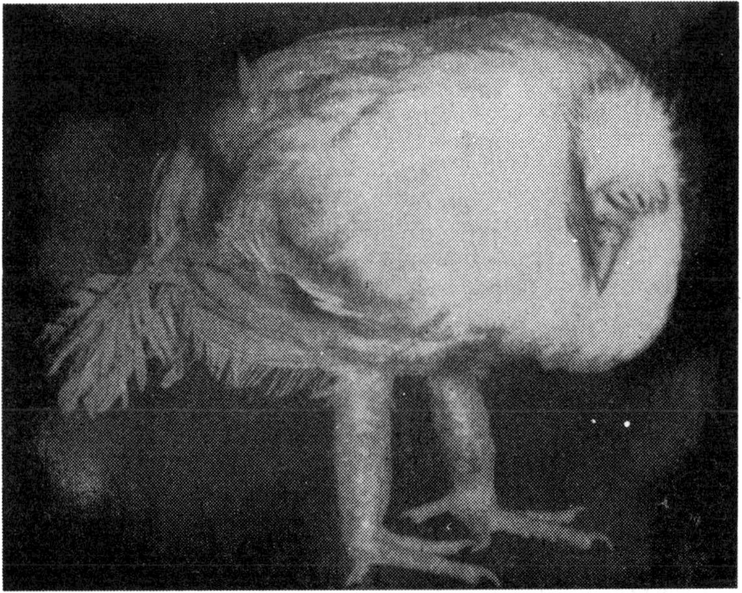

Fig. 4: Marble bone–such enlargement of the shanks and other bones in fowls is caused by osteopetrotic lymphomatosis.

---

[3] Italic numbers in parentheses refer to Literature Cited.

carrying oxygen and nourishment to the different body tissues as well as for revolving waste. Consequently, when the blood shows evidence of disease, there is a general disturbance of the body functions.

Affected birds become anemic–thin, weak and pale. The wattles, comb and skin may become intensely yellow. The blood is often pale and watery. In the late stages of the disease the bird is frequently too weak to stand and this extreme weakness and inactivity are sometimes mistaken for paralysis.

Unlike the other types of this complex, which seldom show progressive changes in the blood cells, the blood types are largely limited to alterations developing within the blood-vessel system. Alterations of the blood or blood circulation may occur which quickly endanger the life of the bird. Frequently great numbers of immature blood cells collect in the smaller blood vessels of the various organs and cause an enlargement which may resemble that in other forms of the leukosis complex. Parts of the bone marrow may be swollen and may vary in colour from dark to white or chalky.

Other Tumors

Various tumors, or neoplasms, of poultry are found in flocks affected with the avian leukosis complex. The tumors are often localized in muscle tissue or are attached to some part of the viscera. Little is known of their origin and though they are frequently classed under the avian leukosis complex, there is some doubt that they are actually connected with it.

Cause of the Avian Leukosis Complex

The cause of the avian leukosis complex with all its various manifestations is not definitely known, even though a great deal of work has been done both by workers concerned with the disease because of its great economic importance to the poultry industry and by those interested in it for the information it might yield on the problem of leukemic diseases in man and other mammals. Most authorities have expressed the opinion that it is caused by a virus or a viruslike agent. The fact that the various types of the avian leukosis complex have been transmitted from bird to bird by various means under suitable conditions strongly suggest that it is of an infectious nature and may spread readily.

Present knowledge would eliminate improper nutrition as a direct cause of the avian leukosis complex. Parasites, such as coccidia and tapeworms, do not cause the disease, although they produce injury that may favour entrance of the leukosis complex agent into the body. Claims that bacteria or their products will induce the disease have not been confirmed. Neither can an unfavourable environment, with faulty ventilation or poor housing, be held responsible.

How is the Disease Transmitted?

To the poultryman probably the most pressing question pertaining to the avian leukosis complex is that of the method of transmission, or spread, of this disease or group of diseases from bird to bird and flock to flock. Effective control measures must await further knowledge of the ways and means by which the disease is spread. Experimental work has shown that it is not difficult to transmit various forms, or types, of the disease by inoculating young birds artificially with blood or material from the organs of diseased birds. It is exceedingly difficult, however, to be sure how the disease is spread under farm and commercial conditions. Under field conditions transmission of the avian leukosis complex would appear to occur in various ways. The observation that the disease seems to have been introduced into clean flocks by hatching eggs or baby chicks from affected sources points to spread through the eggs, possibly in a manner similar to that in which pullorum disease spreads. The fact that the offspring of hens showing various forms of the disease complex sometimes develop the condition at an early age would also favour this possibility.

The fact that the avian leukosis complex has first appeared in a flock after the introduction of birds from flocks where the disease was present suggests spread by contact. Some investigators report transmission of the disease by means of feed contaminated with droppings of affected birds, whereas other workers obtained negative results in similar experiments. In general, however, the common eye, nerve and visceral forms appear to spread more readily under ordinary conditions than the blood, or leukotic, forms. On the other hand, the leukotic forms seem to be more easily transmitted by artificial means, as, for example, by injection of the blood or organs of diseased birds (*50*).

Resistance to the avian leukosis complex increases rapidly with, age, so that special precautions against exposure during the first several months after hatching are justified. Worms, coccidia and other parasites may lower the vitality of the birds and produce, injury through which the disease agent may enter the body tissues. Transmission by mites and ticks, has been suggested and different experiments have yielded both positive and negative results.

Recent observations on the avian leukosis disease complex, as well as on leukotic diseases in other animals, also emphasize the important influence which natural or inherited differences in susceptibility may have on the spread of various infectious and parasitic diseases. Some individuals of a family, or entire families or even strains of birds develop disease after apparently very mild exposure, whereas others do not become affected even when severely exposed. That such resistance may be greatly lowered by unfavourable conditions of housing, handling, or feeding must, however, be fully recognized.

What is Known About Control Measures

Despite the economic importance of the avian leukosis complex and the fact that it has been recognized and studied to some extent for over 20 years, adequate means of control are not known. This situation may be attributed in part to the insidious nature of the disease and in part to the lack of funds, facilities and personnel to study the many aspects of the problem.

The poultry raiser, therefore, cannot at present rely on any definite practical control measures as a protection against serious and recurring losses from the avian leukosis complex. There are, however, two methods, namely, sanitation and breeding, either or both of which hold some promise of being effective.

Importance of Sanitation

Sanitation and hygiene are the keystones of successful management of poultry flocks. Better management is sorely needed on the vast majority of farms where poultry are kept. Poultry will be more thrifty and consequently more profitable, if they are fed a complete diet and housed and yarded in clean, sanitary quarters.

Furthermore, where clean quarters are provided, there will be less chance of exposure to disease agents. Poultry raisers who foster disease through continued neglect and mismanagement not only jeopardize their own interests but maintain a menace to the flocks of those who have adopted sanitary practices.

Sanitation assumes a major role in the transfer of stock from farm to farm and from State to State. The enormous exchange in breeding stock, hatching eggs, baby chicks and live market poultry provides an excellent opportunity for dissemination of disease. Specific management recommendations, though admittedly inadequate in controlling the avian leukosis complex, suggest the adoption of quarantine measures and a minimum exchange of poultry stock.

Distributors of poultry, in any form, must realize that they are handling an animal that is susceptible to a large number of diseases, many of which are infectious and highly contagious. They must see the problem of disease dissemination as it now exists and by united effort attempt to solve it.

Breeding Methods Offer Promise

Careful breeding procedures hold some promise of eventually reducing the incidence of the avian leukosis complex. This may come about in two ways, by mating birds that have the proper hereditary resistant factors and by selecting parents that will not indirectly or by way of the egg transmit the disease to their progeny. Both of these possibilities are supported by sufficient evidence to warrant exhaustive study. Roberts and Card (*47*), reporting on data obtained over a 10 year period on more than 29,000 birds, present evidence that heredity is an important factor in resistance and susceptibility to pullorum disease. Lambert and Knox (*31*) have demonstrated that five generations of selective breeding decreased the mortality from fowl typhoid from 85 to 10 percent. Gildow *et al.* (*18, 19*) reported a reduction of fowl paralysis at the Idaho Experiment Station flock by selective breeding. Marble (*37*) gives data indication a 50 percent decrease in mortality over a 5 year period when selective breeding was practiced.

Asmundson and Biely (2) indicated that there are inherited differences in susceptibility and resistance to fowl paralysis. Patterson and associates (*45*) stated that decided strain differences were found in birds susceptible or resistant to paralysis. These experiments and many others (*3, 10, 11, 32, 36, 57*) with both fowls and mammals indicate that resistance or susceptibility to disease has a genetic basis. It should be emphasized, however, that the absence of disease manifestations does not necessarily indicate genetic resistance, since individual birds or all progeny of certain parents may not have been exposed at all. Such conclusions are warranted only when an adequate number of inoculated controls are available for comparison. It is entirely possible, also, that acquired immunity may account for the failure of many individuals to show manifestations of the disease.

That the egg is a means of pullorum disease transmission has been fully established and the possibility that the avian leukosis complex may be transmitted in a like manner should not be overlooked.

It is recommended that breeding flocks be closed to unrelated birds. The closing of flocks to outside breeding should be practiced more widely than it is. Whenever unproved birds are introduced into a flock, there is great danger of bringing in not only the avian leukosis complex but many other diseases. From a strictly genetic standpoint, uniformity for almost any character will be difficult to attain if birds from new sources are consistently introduced into the breeding pens. The average breeder is reluctant to return to the same source for breeding stock year after year because of the prevalent belief that new blood must be introduced frequently to obtain the best results. This is certainly a misconception on the part of any breeder when large numbers of birds are involved. Marble (37) demonstrated the possibility of reducing losses from disease by using proved blood lines and closing the flocks to outside breeding. Many of the most successful breeders in the United States have maintained closed flocks for years with no loss in either reproductive ability or general health.

The use of elder birds for breeding purposes would appear to have some advantage in that they have at least proved their ability to live for a long time. This procedure would be of little value, however, if the hen were a carrier able to transmit the disease to her progeny. Possibly the better recommendation would be to use hens from families showing high viability, or livability, or from hens that have produced progeny showing high viability.

No Treatment Known

Specific agents or measures for the prevention or treatment of the avian leukosis complex are not known. No feed, vaccine, drug, combination of drugs, or other agent has been found to be of value for the control of this group of diseases. The claim that wheat-germ oil would prevent and cure the nerve type of the leukosis complex has not been confirmed by investigations carried out at a number of experiment stations. Consequently, any claims for direct or specific benefits from medicinal, biological, or other agents or products against the avian leukosis complex must be regarded with extreme caution.

History and Occurrence

A form of transmissible avian leukosis was described by Ellermann and Bang (*7*) as early as 1908. In 1907 Marek (*38*), in Austria, first described a disease in chickens which he called polyneuritis and which is now known as neural lymphomatosis or neurolymphomatosis–the so-called fowl paralysis. The same disease was apparently first described in America by Kaupp in 1921 (*28*). It was subsequently reported from Holland by Van der Walle and Winkler-Junius in 1924 (*55*); from England by Galloway in 1929 (*16*); from Germany by Seifried in 1930 (*49*); and from Japan by Emoto and Miyamoto in 1930 (*8*). Today there is evidence that the avian leukosis complex is widespread throughout the world and that the disease is a serious problem in all areas where the practices of the modern poultry industry (large-scale hatching and distribution) are followed.

Chickens are most commonly and seriously affected by the avian leukosis complex. The disease has been reported also in turkeys, guinea fowl, pheasants and various ornamental birds. Transmission from one species to another seems to occur rarely, if ever. The first 2 to 3 months of life appear to be the period of greatest susceptibility, although exposure to artificial inoculation indicates marked variation in susceptibility among older stock. Great variations, from several days to many months, are observed in the period of incubation (the time from exposure until symptoms or disease changes appear) as well as in the course or duration of the disease, even in the relatively rapidly developing leukosis. In some flocks only a few birds may show signs of the disease, whereas in other flocks a high proportion become affected. Few of the visibly affected individuals recover.

Differences in susceptibility, as determined by the number of affected birds and the time of development of the avian leukosis complex, have been observed among breeds as well as within strains and among families of a breed.

That there are significant sex differences in susceptibility to the avian leukosis complex has not been fully demonstrated.

Scientific Investigations

Scientific study and research dealing with the avian leukosis complex began with the finding of so-called Marek's disease or fowl parallysis in 1907 (*38*) and of a transmissible leukosis by Ellermann and Bang in 1908 (*7*). As already pointed out, the leukosis complex in its various forms was recognized as a major enemy of poultry in various countries before 1930. The malady has attracted the interest and enlisted the energies of many research workers, both abroad and in this country. Progress in the attack on the perplexing problem has, however, been slow and somewhat discouraging.

Observations on various aspects of the problem made by workers in Europe, the United States and Canada and other countries have been largely in agreement. The earlier investigations of the avian leukosis complex in this country were directed chiefly toward study of the nature of the disease and its transmission or spread. Schmeisser (*48*) in 1915 reported artificial transmission of a case of myeloid leukosis to about half the chickens inoculated. May, Tittsler; and Goodner (*39*) gave a preliminary report of field and labouratory findings in so-called fowl paralysis. Doyle (*4, 5*), in spite of negative transmission experiments, suggested the infectious nature of the disease, as well as a relationship between the nerve and eye types. He indicated that the disease was spread by the introduction of stock and through the egg. Pappenheimer and co-workers (*42, 43, 44*) in extensive studies clarified various features of so-called fowl paralysis. They proposed the term "neurolymphomatosis gallinarum" and recognized an apparent relationship between lymphomatosis lesions in the nerves and in other tissues. The disease was transmitted by injection with diseased nerves. No relation was found between, paralysis and infestation with coccidia and intestinal worms. Patterson and associates (*45*) presented evidence of the spread of the avian leukosis complex by means of manure and contaminated litter. Work at other stations Ohio (*29*), Idaho (*18, 19*), South Carolina (*1*), Illinois (*54*) and Connecticut (26)) tended to confirm this observation. Ratcliffe and Stubbs (*46*) failed to transmit leukosis by mosquitoes and mites. Johnson (*24*) concluded that mites could carry the disease from affected to healthy birds and that it might be mechanically transmitted during the process of vaccination against fowl pox.

The work of Furth (*12, 13, 14*), Furth and Breedis (*15*), Stubbs (*51*) and Stubbs and Furth (*52, 53*), dealing with various manifestations of the disease grouped as the avian leukosis complex, indicated differences among strains of the agent or agents causing leukosis, as well as between the agents responsible for leukosis and lymphomatosis. This view was supported by the findings of Feldman and Olson (*9, 10*) Olson (*40, 41*), Fenstermacher (*11*) and Jungherr (*25, 26, 27*). The Iowa workers [Patterson and associates (*45*), Lee and associates (*33, 34*)], as well as Johnson (*22, 23*), hold the view that all manifestations of the avian leukosis complex are associated with a common causative agent. Wilcke and co-workers (*58*) found that cod-liver oil, yeast, green feed, iodine and various ratios and amounts of calcium and phosphorus had no effect on the incidence or course of the disease.

Observations on the influence of heredity on susceptibility and resistance to the avian leukosis complex have already been alluded to. This phase of the problem is now receiving much attention.

The recent work of Durant and McDougle (*6*) suggests the importance of egg transmission and the almost continuous infectivity of the blood of chicks from clinically affected dams. Lee reported in 1940[4] that affected hens apparently are much more likely to transmit the disease through the egg than are diseased males. Gibbs (*17*), Kirschbaum and Stern (*30*), Hall and associates (*20*) and Brandly and Cottral[5] were able to induce manifestations of the avian leukosis complex by inoculating incubating chick embryos or their membranes with the blood, tissues and extracts of diseased birds.

Though the findings of these and other investigations have added materially to the information on the disease or diseases designated as the avian leukosis complex, it is clear that much additional information is desirable and necessary. Some of the lack

---

4 In a paper presented at seventy-sixth annual meeting of the American Veterinary Medical Association.

5 Unpublished data, 1940.

of agreement in work and opinions may be ascribed to difficulties peculiar to the study of diseases with long incubation or developmental periods, irregular manifestations and undetermined causes. Likewise, studies with hosts or birds of unknown genetic background magnify the difficulties. These problems obviously demand a more comprehensive and coordinated programme supported by proper facilities and suitable personnel if they are to be successfully attacked.

A Coordinated Programme of Research Begun

In view of the seriousness of the poultry-disease situation as represented by the avian leukosis complex and various other conditions, recommendations were drawn up during1937 in a conference of 25 directors of experiment stations in the North-central and North-eastern States. The Secretary of the United States Department of Agriculture was subsequently petitioned to establish a regional labouratory for the improvement of viability in poultry. The Regional Poultry Research Labouratory was approved and was established at East Lansing, Mich., March 25, 1938. Its work is done in close and active co-operation with that in each of the 25 North-central and North-eastern States and that of the Animal Disease Station, Beltsville, Md., where investigation of this disease has been carried on for several years. In this research programme, experiment station workers and the Regional Poultry Research Labouratory Staff are collabourating in the investigation of various ways and means for the control of the avian leukosis complex. Such collabouration will eliminate needless duplication of effort and at the same time provide the labouratory with active and advisory assistance.

Of the 31 State experiment stations in the United States which have undertaken studies of the avian leukosis complex, 21 are in the group of States designated as the major region of the Regional Poultry Research Labouratory programme. Besides these experiment stations, numerous other institutions in various States are investigating the avian leukosis complex particularly as it relates to leukemia and similar conditions found in other species, including man.

At the present time, 10 States within the major region have co-operative projects with the Labouratory. These States are conducting work either in combination or separately on various phases of pathology, breeding and nutrition.

Investigations Under Way

The work project of the regional programme has four aspects: Genetic and physiologic, management, nutritional and pathologic. Because there are neither funds nor facilities available to undertake at the start all the phases of the research that need attention, the genetics and physiology and the pathology (the study of the nature of the disease itself) will receive first attention.

The Genetic Approach

A genetic approach to this problem calls for the formation of families inherently resistant or susceptible to fowl leukosis and possessing to a marked degree characters of general economic value (56). Though susceptible families would be of little economic importance, their genetic value would be great, for without such lines the mode of inheritance of resistance and the influence of the environment would be difficult to determine. In addition, susceptible non-carrier stocks are necessary for pathologic studies, including epizoology (the study of the disease as an epidemic among animals), immunization and various non-genetic control methods.

Careful consideration was given to the selection of birds to be used for experimental purposes at the Regional Labouratory. A survey of breeding stock in the United States indicated that it was possible to obtain from widely separated geographic regions many strains of Single Comb White Leghorns about the viability and production of which much was known. The White Leghorn was therefore selected as the most suitable material for the research on fowl paralysis.

In the spring of 1939, more than 1,000 hatching eggs were introduced from each of 10 different White Leghorn flocks. Upon hatching, the chicks were divided into two groups. One group, unexposed to the avian leukosis complex, used as a control, was confined in strictly quarantined houses on the west, or control, side of the plant. The other group was sub-divided into an inoculated group and a non-inoculated, pen-contact group, which was confined in the same pens with the inoculated chicks and quarantined in similar houses on the east, or infection, side or unit of the plant. All the chicks, except those from one flock which were subsequently discarded, were of known ancestry. This fact permitted a distribution of chicks from the same dam to both control and inoculated groups. The inoculated birds were to provide an estimate of the resistance or susceptibility of their unexposed sibs (sisters and brothers).

Only birds from the non-inoculated control units were to be used for breeding purposes. It was decided to close the entire flock to all outside breeding and to attempt a breeding programme which would as quickly as possible segregate the birds with the greatest number of desirable characters and those with the fewest. In a breeding experiment with a closed flock, no inherited trait can be incorporated into a group of birds except for possible mutations unless the genes exist in the original foundation stock. This emphasizes the importance of starting with suitable material.

One of the main objectives of the breeding programme is to segregate birds resistant or susceptible to fowl paralysis as quickly as possible while sacrificing valuable economic characters as little as possible. On the basis of incomplete family performance, therefore, birds of the original 1939 population within families showing the most resistance and those within families showing the most susceptibility were mated to obtain a 1940 population. The chicks hatched in 1940 were divided into inoculated and control groups as in the case of the 1939 population.

Pathology Phase

The pathology programme includes studies planned or under way on methods of diagnosis, both before and after the appearance of symptoms; possible means of detecting carriers; means of transmission, including the role that parasites, bacteria and other agents may play; the nature, properties and tissue distribution of the causative agent or agents; embryo and chick susceptibility; the mechanism of acquired immunity; and the development and improvement of experimental methods and procedures for the study of the avian leukosis complex.

The initial study at the Laboratory was projected jointly toward a study of the susceptibility and resistance of the 10 strains of chickens on the one hand and on the other, of the properties of several strains or causative agents of the avian leukosis complex.

Extensive examination of all the birds that developed disease during the course of the experimental work was recognized as necessary in order to make accurate diagnoses. The data collected from the examinations indicate the nature and distribution of the lesions. The value of such information from the practical as well as the experimental standpoint is apparent.

The fact that a very high percentage of birds less than 3 weeks of age (approximately 1,700) inoculated in April and May 1939 with lymphomatosis material from two different sources developed the disease is not particularly significant. Under the conditions that prevailed, however, the occurrence of the disease among each of the 10 strains of the un-inoculated, or control, population would tend to incriminate egg transmission of the avian leukosis complex as important. In this connection it is pointed out that only hatching eggs representing the 10 different strains were brought onto the Labouratory premises. Live poultry and other birds as well as animals and human beings, from the outside were excluded. Furthermore, all buildings were under quarantine and strict sanitary precautions were followed. The caretakers were limited to the separate units and required to change clothing and footwear before going from one unit to another and other rigid quarantine measures were observed. Complete confinement of all birds has been practiced since the beginning of the experiment. Despite all these precautions, cases of the avian leukosis complex began to appear among birds in the west or control unit of the Labouratory as early as 40 days after the first hatching of eggs from the original 10 strains of White Leghorns. The disease did not appear any earlier in the birds in the east or infection unit, even though approximately two-thirds of the latter stock were inoculated at an early age with the blood of birds showing disease changes characteristic of some form of the avian leukosis complex. Furthermore, the mortality from the avian leukosis complex among the 1939 population was not significantly less in the birds in the control unit than in the birds reared in contact with the inoculated stock.

The results obtained, under strict quarantine and sanitary measures, may be regarded as satisfactory despite the appearance of the avian leukosis complex among the control birds, because no other diseases or parasites, with the exception of sporadic cases of coccidiosis, have been found on the premises. The first outbreak of coccidiosis, in several houses and among both controls and inoculated birds, occurred in November 1939, 8 months after the work was started. The manner in which coccidiosis first appeared suggests contamination by way of feed or litter, or both.

In serial-passage[6] experiments, the inoculation of different groups of chicks with lymphomatotic material from widely separated sources has consistently reproduced both nerve and visceral types of the disease. One of these strains of inoculum has associated with it the bone changes termed "osteopetrosis." The bone changes have been seen in about half the chicks inoculated with that particular strain, or agent. Furthermore, when the material was inoculated into incubating eggs, the resulting chicks showed about the same percentage of bone changes as the birds inoculated after hatching. Osteopetrosis has not been seen in uninoculated birds kept continuously in the same pens with affected individuals for long periods. Another of the strains of material used for inoculation in the serial-passage work has induced a high percentage of blood, or leukosis, cases. In the serial-passage experiments with strains showing osteopetrosis and leukosis, respectively, the nerve and visceral forms of the disease, were also manifested. This might be accepted as proof of the capacity of a particular strain to induce all manifestations and types of the disease complex if it were not for the development of similar numbers of cases of nerve and visceral types of the disease in uninjected control birds.

These observations do not clarify the question whether all types of disease classed within the avian leukosis complex are due to one causative agent or whether each type or a combination of types is caused by a separate and distinct agent. The observations on the source, or strain, of the material used for inoculation do, however, emphasize clearly that progress on this entire problem will depend to a large extent on securing disease-free stock for experimental purposes. In order to identify the agent or agents causing the avian leukosis complex and to measure the resistance or susceptibility of birds, there must be reasonable assurance that the disease has not been introduced either by way of the egg or by any other means. This phase of the problem, therefore, is being studied intensively.

---

[6] Serial passage is passage of the disease from bird to bird by artificial inoculation of a healthy chick with tissues from an individual affected with the disease.

Other Phases of the Investigation

Many other phases of the problem presented by the avian leukosis complex have been outlined as a part of the long-time labouratory programme. Some work that has been outlined cannot be undertaken at present because of lack of facilities and personnel. Other parts of the programme must await the results of investigations under way in other branches of science before they can be approached properly and to the best advantage.

Poultry management factors that demand study and clarification include (1) the value of sanitary procedures and; (2) the time required for the infection present in contaminated areas and premises to die out.

Nutritional aspects of the problem to be studied embrace the effect of diet on the incidence of the avian-leukosis complex in stock of known genetic background.

Literature Cited

(1) ANDERSON, G.W., RINGROSE, R.C. and MORGAN, C.L. (1937). A STUDYOF SO-CALLED FOWL PARALYSIS. S.C. Agr. Expt. Sta. Ann. Rpt. 50: 73.

(2) ASMUNDSON, V.S. and BIELY, JACOB (1932). INHERITANCE OF RESISTANCE TO FOWL PARALYSIS (NEUROLYMPHOMATOSIS GALLINARUM). I. DIFFERENCES IN SUSCEPTIBILITY. Canad. Jour. Res. 6: 171-176.

(3) BIELY, JACOB, PALMER, ELVIRA and ASMUNDSON, V.S. (1932). INHERITANCE OF RESISTANCE TO FOWL PARALYSIS (NEUROLYMPHOMATOSIS GALLINARUM). II. ON A SIGNIFICANT DIFFERENCE IN THE INCIDENCE OF FOWL PARALYSIS IN TWO GROUPS OF CHICKS. Canad. Jour.Res.6: 374-380, illus.

(4) DOYLE, L.P. (1926). NEURITIS IN CHICKENS. Amer. Vet. Med. Assoc. Jour. 68: 622-630, illus.

(5) ____(1928). NEURITIS OR PARALYSIS IN CHICKENS. Amer. Vet. Med. Assoc. Jour. 72: 585-587.

(6) DURANT, A.J. and McDOUGLE, H.C. (1939). STUDIES ON THE ORIGIN AND TRANSMISSION OF FOWL PARALYSIS (NEUROLYMPHOMATOSIS) BY BLOOD INOCULATION. Mo. Agr. Expt. Sta. Res. Bul. 304, 23 pp., illus.

(7) ELLERMANN, V. and BANG, O. (1908). EXPERIMENTELLE LEUKAMIE BEI HUHNERN. Centbl. f. Bakt. [etc.] Originale (I) 46: 595-600, illus.

(8) EMOTO, O. and MIYAMOTO, K. (1930). STUDIES ON THE FOWL PARALYSIS. Jap. Soc. Vet. Sci. Jour. 9: 309-325, illus.

(9) FELDMAN, WILLIAM H. and OLSON, CARL, JR. (1933). THE PATHOLOGY OF SPONTANEOUS LEUKOSIS OF CHICKENS. Amer. Vet. Med. Assoc. Jour. 82: 875-900, illus.

(10) _____and OLSON, CARL JR. (1934). LEUKOSIS OF THE COMMON CHICKEN. Amer. Vet. Med. Assoc. Jour. 84: 488-498.

(11) FENSTERMACHER, R. (1936). LYMPHOCYTOMA AND FOWL PARALYSIS. Amer. Vet. Med. Assoc. Jour. 88: 600-613.

(12) FURTH, J. (1931). ERYTHROLEUKOSIS AND THE ANEMIAS OF THE FOWL. Arch. Path. 12: 1-30, illus.

(13) _____(1933). LYMPHOMATOSIS, MYELOMATOSIS AND ENDOTHELIONA OF CHICKENS CAUSED BY A FILTERABLE AGENT. I. TRNSMISSION EXPERIMENTS. Jour. Expt. Med. 58: 253-275.

(14) _____(1936). THE RELATION OF LEUKOSIS TO SARCOMA OF CHICKENS. II. MIXED OSTEOCHONDROSARCOMA AND LYMPHOMATOSIS (STAIN 12). Jour. Expt. Med. 63: 127-143, illus. III. SARCOMATA OF STRAINS 11 AND 15 AND THEIR RELATION TO LEUKOSIS. Jour. Expt. Med. 63: 145-155, illus.

(15) _____and BREEDIS, CHARLES (1935). LYMPHOMATOSIS IN RELATION TO FOWL PARALYSIS. Arch. Path. 20: 379-428, illus.

(16) GALLOWAY, A.I. (1929). DISCUSSION ON ENCEPHALO-MYELITIS OF MAN AND ANIMALS. Joint Discuss. No. 8, Roy. Soc.-Ked. Proc. 22: 1167-1171.

(17) GIBBS, CHARLES S. (1936). OBSERVATIONS AND EXPERIMENTS WITH NEUROLYMPHOMATOSIS AND THE LEUKOTIC DISEASES. Mass. Agr. Expt. Sta. Bull. 337, 31 pp., illus.

(18) GILDOW, E. M., WILLIAMS, J.K. and LAMPMAN, C.E. (1936). THE TRANSMISSION OF FOWL PARALYSIS (LYMPHOKATOSIS). Poultry Sci. 15: 244-248.

(19) _____WILLIAMS, J.K. and LAMPKAN, C.E. (1940). THE TRANSMISSION OF AND RESISTANCE TO FOWL PARALYSIS (LYMPHOMATOSIS). Idaho Agr. Expt. Sta. Bull. 235, 22 pp., illus.

(20) HALL, W.J., BEAN, C.W. and POLLARD, MORRIS L. (1940). PRELIMINARY REPORT ON THE PROPAGATION OF THE FOWL-LEUCOSIS VIRUS ON CHICK EMBRYOS BY INTRAVENOUS INOCULATION. Amer. Vet. Med. Assoc. Jour. 97: 247.

(21) HAMILTON, C.M. and SAWYER, C.E. (1939). TRANSMISSION OF ERYTHROLEUKOSIS IN YOUNG CHICKENS. Poultry Sci. 18; 388-393.

(22) JOHNSON, E.P. (1932). A STUDY OF LYKPHOKATOSIS OF FOWLS (FOWL PARALYSIS). Va. Agr. Expt. Sta. Tech. Bull. 44, 22 pp., illus.

(23) _____(1934). THE ETIOLOGY AND HISTOGENESIS OF LEUCOSIS AND LYMPHOMATOSIS OF FOWLS. Va. Agr. Expt. Sta. Tech. Bull. 56, 32 pp., illus.

(24) _____(1937). TRANSMISSION OF FOWL LEUKOSIS. Poultry Sci. 16: 255-260.

(25) JUNGHEBR, ERWIN (1935). THE ETIOLOGIC AND DIAGNOSTIC ASPECTS OF THE FOWL PARALYSIS PROBLEM. Amer. Vet. Med. Assoc. Jour. 86: 424-432, illus.

(26) _____(1937). STUDIES ON FOWL PARALYSIS. 2. TRANSMISSION EXPERIMENTS. Conn., (Storrs) Agr. Expt. Sta. Bull. 218, 47 pp., illus.

(27) _____and LANDAUER, W. (1938). STUDIES ON FOWL PARALYSIS. 3. A CONDITION RESEMBLING OSTEOPETROSIS (MARBLE BONE) IN THE COMMON FOWL. Conn. (Storrs) Agr. Expt. Sta. Bull. 222, 34pp., illus.

(28) KAUPP, B.F. (1921). PARALYSIS OF THE DOMESTIC FOWL. Amer. Assoc. Instr. and Invest. Poultry Husb. Jour. 7: 25-31, illus.

(29) KENNARD, D.C. and CHAMBERLIN, V.D. (1934). PULLET MORTALITY. Ohio Agr. Expt. Sta. Bimo; Bull. 19 (169); 137-142, illus.

(30) KIRSCHBAUM, ARTHUR and STERN, KURT G. (1940). LEUKEMIA IN THE FOWL FOLLOWING INOCULATION OF NON-CELLULAR AGENT OBTAINED BY ULTRACENTRIFUGATION OF LEUKEMIC BONE MRROW EXTRACT AND PLASMA. Anat. Rec. 76, Sup. 2 (Abstracts of papers), p. 37.

(31) LAMBERT, W.V. and KNOX, C.W. (1932). SELECTION FOR RESISTANCE TO FOWL TYPHOID IN THE CHICKEN WITH REFERENCE TO ITS INHERITANCE. Iowa Agr. Expt. Sta. Res. Bull. 153: 261-295, illus.

(32) LAMPMAN, C.E. (1937). FLOCKS ESTABLISH RESISTANCE TO FOWL PARALYSIS. Idaho Agr. Expt. Sta. Ann. Rpt. 1936 (Bull. 221); 43-44.

(33) LEE, C.D., WILCKE, H.L., MURRAY, CHAS. and HENDERSON, E.W. (1937). FOWL LEUCOSIS. Amer. Vet. Med. Assoc. Jour. 91: 146-162.

(34) _____WILCKE, H.L., MURRAY. CHAS and HENDERSON, E.W. (1937). FOWL LEUKOSIS. Jour. Infect. Dis. 61: [1]-20.

(35) McCLARY, C.F. and UPP, CHAS. W. (1939). IS PARALYSIS OF FOWLS, AS MANIFESTED BY IRITIS, TRANSMITTED., THROUGH THE EGG Poultry Sci. 18: 210-219, illus.

(36) MADSEN, D.E. (1937). THE EFFECT OF IRITIS OF BREEDING HENS ON THEIR PROGENY. Poultry Sci. 16: 393-397.

(37) MARBLE, D.R. (1939). BREEDING POULTRY FOR VIABILITY. Pa. Agr. Expt. Sta. Bull. 377, 38 pp., illus.

(38) MAREK, J. (1907). MULTIPLE NERVENENTZUNDUNG (POLYNEURITIS) BEI HUHNERN. Deut. Tierarztl. Wchnsch. 15: [417]-421, illus.

(39) MAY, HENRY G., TITTSLER, RALPH P. and GOODNER, KENNETH (1925). FIELD OBSERVATIONS AND LABOURATORY FINDINGS IN PARALYSIS OF THE DOMESTIC FOWL. R.I. Expt. Sta. Bull. 202, 18 pp., illus.

(40) OLSON, CARL, JR. (1936). A STUDY OF TRANSMISSIBLE FOWL LEUKOSIS. Amer. Vet. Med. Assoc. Jour. 89: 681-705, illus.

(41) _____(1940). TRANSMISSIBLE FOWL LEUKOSIS. A REVIEW OF THE LITERATURE. Mass. Agr. Expt. Sta. Bull. 370, 48 pp.

(42) PAPPENHEIMER, ALVIN M., DUNN, LESLIE A. and GONE, VERNON (1926). A STUDY OF FOWL PARALYSIS (NEUROLYMPHOMATOSIS GALLINARUM). Conn. (Storrs) Agr. Expt. Sta. Bull. 143, pp. 183-290, illus.

(43) _____DUNN, LESLIE C. and GONE, VERNON (1929). STUDIES ON FOWL PARALYSIS (NEUROLYMPHOMATOSIS GALLINARUM). I. CLINICAL FEATURES AND PATHOLOGY. Jour. Expt. Med. 49: 63-86, illus.

(44) _____DUNN, LESLIE C. and SEIDLIN, S.M. (1929). STUDIES ON FOWL PARALYSIS (NEUROLYMPHOMATOSIS GALLINARUM). II. TRANSMISSION EXPERIMENTS. Jour. Expt. Med. 49: 87-102.

(45) PATTERSON, F.D., WILOKE, H.L., MURRAY, CHAS. and HENDERSON, E.W. (1932). SO-CALLED RANGE PARALYSIS OF CHICKENS. Amer. Vet. Med. Assoc. Jour. 81: 747-767, illus.

(46) RATCLIFFE, HERBERT L. and STUBBS, E.L. (1935). ATTEMPTS TO TRANSMIT CHICKEN LEUKOSIS BY MOSQUITOES AND BY MITES. Jour. Infect. Dis. 56: [301]-304.

(47) ROBERTS, ELMER and CARD, L.E. (1935). INHERITANCE OF RESISTANCE TO BACTERIAL INFECTION IN ANIMALS. Ill. Agr. Expt. Sta. Bull. 419: 465-493, illus.

(48) SCHMEISSER, HARRY C. (1915). SPONTANEOUS AND EXPERIMENTAL LEUKEMIA OF THE FOWL. Jour. Expt. Med. 22; 820-838.

(49) SEIFRIED, OSKAB (1930). INFEKTIOSE PARALYSE REI HUHNERN. Arch. f. Wiss. u. Prakt. Tierheilk. 62: [209]-222, illus.

(50) STUBBS, E.L. (1933). THE RELATION OF AGE, BREED AND SPECIES TO SUSCEPTIBILITY TO TRANSMISSIBLE LEUCOSIS OF CHICKENS. Jour. Amer. Vet. Med. Assoc. 82: 232-242.

(51) _____(1988). FOWL LEUKOSIS. Amer. Vet. Med. Assoc. Jour. 92: 73-82.

(52) _____and FUBTH, J. (1981). TRANSMISSION EXPERIMENTS WITH LEUCOSIS OF FOWLS. Jour. Expt. Med. 53: 269-276.

(53) _____and FURTH, J. (1935). THE RELATION OF LEUKOSIS TO SARCOMA OF CHICKENS. I. SARCOMA AND ERYTHROLEUKOSIS (STRAIN 13). Jour. Expt. Med. 61: 593-615, illus.

(54) THORP, FRANK, JR. and GRAHAM, ROBERT (1936). TRANSMISSION STUDIES IN LEUCEMIA. Vet. Med. 31: 82-85, illus.

(55) WALLE, N. VAN DER and WINKLER-JUNIUS, E. (1924). DE NEURITIS-EPIZOÖTIE BIJ KIPPEN TE BARNEVELD IN 1921. Tijdschr. v. Vergelijk. Geneesk. 10: 34-50, illus. [In Dutch. English summary, pp. 46-47.]

(56) WATERS, NELSON F. and BYWATERS, JAMES H. (1941). THE PROPOSED BREEDING PROGRAMME OF THE REGIONAL POULTRY RESEARCH LABOURATORY. Poultry Sci. 20: 221-223.

(57) WILOKE, H.L., LEE, C.D. and MURRAY, CHARLES (1938). SUSCEPTIBILITY AND RESISTANCE OF SOME STRAINS OF CHICKENS TO FOWL LEUCOSIS. Poultry Sci. 17: 58-66, illus.

(58) _____PATTERSON, F.D., HENDERSON, E.W. and MURRAY, CHARLES (1933). THE EFFECT OF THE RATION UPON THE INCIDENCE OF SO-CALLED RANGE PARALYSIS. Poultry Sci. 12: 226-232.

Chapter 3

RESPIRATORY DISEASES OF CHICKENS AND TURKEYS

W.J. Hall [1]

[1] *W.J. Hall is Veterinarian, Animal Disease Station, Bureau of Animal Industry.*

Every year poultry producers incur heavy losses from respiratory diseases in their flocks. Here is a careful account of the causes, symptoms, diagnosis, treatment and prevention of these maladies.

Several respiratory diseases of fowls cause major losses to the poultry industry throughout the country. These losses, which usually occur in the fall or winter, after the expense of rearing the chickens has been incurred and when replacement is difficult and costly, can be prevented only by constant vigilance and attention to management and traffic in fowls. In come cases and under certain circumstances, preventive vaccination may be helpful.

The most important diseases affecting the respiratory tract of chickens are infectious laryngotracheitis, infectious bronchitis,. and infectious coryza. Other diseases that may produce respiratory symptoms are fowl pox, pullorum disease, aspergillosis, fowl paralysis, gapes and occasionally infestation by air-sac mites. In fowl pox, hollow casts or linings of cheeselike pus may form an obstruction in the larynx to the free interchange of air. In pullorum disease and in aspergillosis abscesses may be so numerous as to interfere seriously with the oxygenation of the blood. Gapeworms sometimes collect in such numbers as to restrict breathing. In some cases of fowl paralysis the nerve supply to the respiratory apparatus is damaged, causing difficulty in breathing. Gasping, or gapes, is the common symptom in all the disease conditions that interfere with breathing.

Infectious Laryngotracheitis

Infectious laryngotracheitis has been variously called infectious bronchitis, infectious tracheitis, tracheolaryngitis, chicken "flu," and Canadian "flu." The name "infectious laryngotracheitis," suggested in 1930, has finally been generally adopted as being the most suitable.

The disease is found in all parts of the United States and in Canada, England, Germany, Hawaii and Australia. Chickens of all ages, from baby chicks to mature fowls, are effected.

Respiratory diseases resembling laryngotracheitis were noted by poultry feeders at the beginning of the century. The mortality was comparatively low in these outbreaks. The affected birds were known as wheezers or callers and removing them from the flock was effective in preventing serious losses. It was not until about 1920, however, that the disease was described by poultry pathologists.

In 1930 and 1931 the causative agent was definitely established as a filtrable virus[2] (*1, 3, 14, 15*).[3] The virus is quickly destroyed by disinfectants such as 3 percent solution of liquor cresolis compositis, 1-percent lye solution, or 5 percent carbolic acid, as well as by 7 hours of exposure to direct sunlight. Under favourable conditions it may survive on contaminated premises as long as 3 months. In dead birds the virus does not survive the decomposition of the carcass (*27*).

The mucous membrane lining the respiratory tract of the fowl is the principal tissue affected. In the acute form of the disease the mucous membrane of the larynx and trachea is the site of the

---

[2] A filtrable virus is a disease-producing agent so small that it will pass through fine porcelain bacteria-retaining filters, and it is invisible even with the aid of a microscope.

[3] Italic numbers in parentheses refer to Literature Cited.

principal tissue changes. In the milder subacute or chronic form the mucous membrane of the conjunctivae (the lining of the eyelids) and of the nasal and ocular sinuses may also become affected. The secretions of the respiratory tract are the richest source of virus. It has also been reported in the spleens and livers of infected birds (2).

The disease comes on suddenly. In the acute form the course is usually rapid, the affected bird recovering or dying within a week or less. In less virulent (subacute) outbreaks the disease may be localized in the eyes and adjacent sinuses and the course may be prolonged to 2 or 3 weeks. The incubation period (the time between exposure to the disease and the appearance of symptoms) in the acute form has been stated to be 3 to 10 days and in natural outbreaks 7 to 12 days (*20, 21*).

A tentative diagnosis of the disease may be made by noting the principal symptoms and lesions (tissue changes), but in order to make a positive diagnosis differentiating the condition from others that resemble it, cross-immunity tests may be necessary.

The outstanding symptom of laryngotracheitis is gasping. On inhaling, the head is extended upward with mouth wide open. (Fig. 1, *A*) and on expiration the head is retracted on the breast, with the mouth closed (Fig. 1, *B*). This series of motions is repeated with, each breath. The gasping is interrupted occasionally by coughing, followed by shaking of the head in an endeavour to rid the nose and mouth of the mucus, blood and pus brought up in coughing. Respiration is usually accompanied by a variety of noises, rattling, wheezing and sometimes loud cries. The breathing noises are caused by partial obstructions of the respiratory passages with exudates, or discharges, of blood-stained mucus and pus.

Laryngotracheitis is usually mild in young chicks and may be wrongly diagnosed as a cold.

Cross-immunity tests cannot safely be carried out on the farm. If labouratory service cannot be secured to conduct such tests, a tentative diagnosis may be made by careful observations of the following principal characteristics of laryngotracheitis: Sudden onset and rapid spread; rapid course–nearly all deaths occur within a week and are due to suffocation; gasping respiration; coughing up blood-stained exudate; and the confinement of the lesions in early cases to the larynx and trachea, which contains a variable amount of mucus, pus and blood.

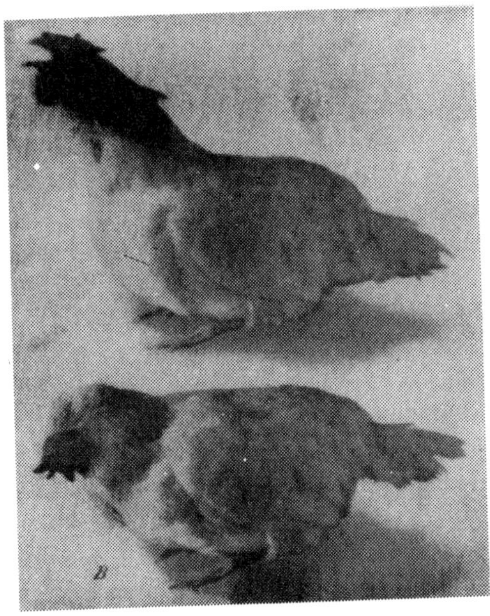

Fig 1: A hen with a severe case of laryngotracheitis, showing *A*: attitude during inspiration, *B*: attitude during expiration. (Courtesy of the Division of Veterinary Science, California Agricultural Experiment Station.)

A cross-immunity test may be conducted as follows: Tracheal exudate is collected from a bird in with suspected laryngotracheitis by inserting a sterile cotton swab into the trachea. The exudate on the swab is then immediately transferred to the trachea of a normal susceptible bird (one that has never been exposed to any respiratory disease). In the same manner a bird that has been immunized to infectious laryngotracheitis by cloacal vaccination (described later) is inoculated. If the susceptible bird develops the disease while the immune bird remains well, there is strong evidence that the disease is laryngotracheitis. If both birds develop a respiratory disease as a result of the inoculation of the unknown agent, the disease is not infectious laryngotracheitis but may be infectious bronchitis, which is caused by a filtrable virus that is distinct from the standpoint of immunity, from the virus of laryngotracheitis.

The principal tissue changes in a typical acute outbreak are located in the larynx and trachea, as the name of the disease indicates. Severe inflammation of the mucous membrane lining these organs produces a great increase in the amount of mucus discharge, which becomes blood-stained from capillary hemorrhages and later is thickened and yellowish. As the discharge dries on the walls of the trachea and larynx it may form a hollow cast, or false membrane. As more mucus dries within this cast the opening is gradually narrowed until breathing becomes difficult or impossible and death results from suffocation. In other cases, suffocation is caused by the formation of a cheesy pus in the larynx.

In mild cases such complications may ensue as swelling and exudation in the nasal passages, eyelids and adjacent sinuses, which are clinically indistinguishable from the so-called roup, or coryza. In other cases the disease may terminate in pneumonia or bronchitis.

Losses from this disease are due not only to a relatively high mortality but also to a marked drop in egg production and a greatly increased number of unthrifty birds. The death losses vary from few or none in young chicks in warm weather up to 70 percent in heavy birds in high production in cold weather. One survey showed that losses from the drop in egg production following an outbreak may amount to one-fourth the loss from mortality.

The most important method of spread is the carrier bird. A bird that recovers from the disease is immune but becomes a carrier for life. Although such a bird may appear healthy, the exudate from its respiratory tract is highly virulent to susceptible birds. If carrier birds are retained in a flock, each new crop of chicks may be infected and the disease thus perpetuated. It may also be spread from flock to flock by means of contaminated crates and probably also by contaminated clothing of caretakers, feed bags and utensils.

The part played by wild birds and vermin in disseminating the disease has not been definitely established, but they should be excluded from contact with poultry as much as possible.

That the virus of laryngotracheitis is not transmitted by or through the egg is fairly well established (5).

Various chemicals and disinfectants have been recommended for the treatment of laryngotracheitis by spraying, vaporization and administration in the feed and drinking water, but controlled experimental tests have shown that they are of little value in the cure of this disease.

The best methods of prevention are sanitation and vaccination. Visitors should be excluded from the poultry quarters as much as possible.

Traffic in birds should be reduced to a minimum.

Shipping crates should be disinfected before being returned to poultry quarters.

In 1932 Hudson and Beaudette (*18*) discovered that application of the virus of laryngotracheitis to the mucous membrane of the cloaca (vent) and bursa Fabricius (a gland opening into the cloaca) produced only a local reaction lasting about 10 days and characterized by swelling and redness and the formation of a small amount of pus at the site of vaccination. After recovery, the bird was immune to the disease. This technique proved to be a satisfactory method of vaccination (*4*).

Laryngotracheitis vaccine is prepared from the tracheal exudate, or discharge, of infected fowls. This material, consisting of mucus, blood, pus and cast-off cells from the mucous membrane, is dried under vacuum, ground to a fine powder and then mixed with a measured amount of 50 percent glycerine immediately before use. A more recent method of producing the vaccine is the propagation of the virus on developing chick embryos, in which the virus may be grown free of bacteria.

The vaccine is applied to the mucous membrane of the cloaca by means of several vigorous strokes of a stiff bristle brush until redness or a slight hemorrhage is produced. After 5 days the bird is examined for a vaccination reaction, or take, evidenced by swelling and redness of the mucous membrane of the cloaca (Fig. 2). If no take is apparent the bird must be revaccinated, as such birds, except an occasional one that possesses natural immunity, may otherwise develop the disease in the trachea. Birds successfully vaccinated are immune for life. For the first 10 or 12 days after vaccination, virus may be eliminated in the droppings and during that time a vaccinated bird is a potential source of danger to birds in the flock that were not successfully vaccinated. After that period however, the vaccinated bird is not only immune but does not become a virus carrier, as does one that has recovered from a natural attack of the disease.

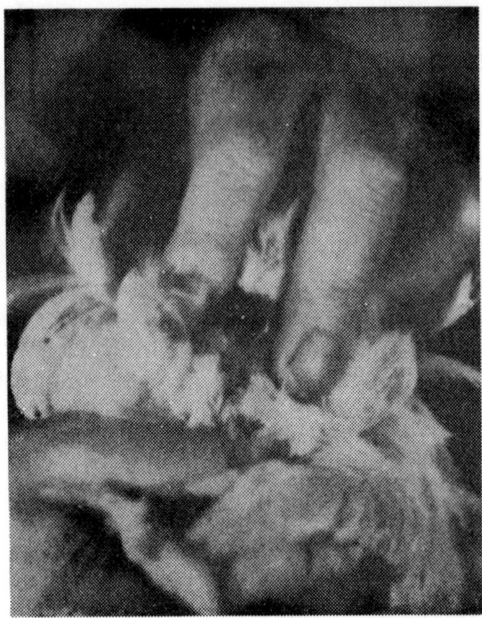

Fig. 2: Cloacal mucous membrane of a chicken, swollen and red as the result of vaccination for laryngotracheltis. This reaction indicates a take, which is followed by immunity. (Courtesy of the Division of Veterinary Science, California Agricultural Experiment Station).

Vaccination against laryngotracheitis is usually recommended only under the following circumstances:

(1) When the disease is prevalent in the immediate neighbourhood and when it occurs from year to year in the pullets owing to the presence in the flock of carriers from previous outbreaks;

(2) When birds, usually males, are brought into the flock from outside sources where exposure was probable; and

(3) In outbreaks in large flocks where the disease is confined to one pen. In the last case, the birds in the other pens may be saved by vaccination if it is done promptly.

Where the disease was present the year before, chicks should be vaccinated when 2 to 3 months old. At that age they may be vaccinated at the same time against pox.

Where no laryngotracheitis exists in the neighbourhood and there is little if any chance of exposure of the flock to the disease vaccination should not be practiced, since after the vaccine, which is a live virus, is introduced into a flock, annual vaccination may be necessary in order to protect each new crop of pullets from possible carriers.

Infectious Bronchitis

Infectious bronchitis is a respiratory disease primarily of young chicks. It is immunologically distinct–that is, infection with one disease does not create immunity against the other–from infectious laryngotracheitis and infectious coryza. It is sometimes called gasping disease of chicks.

First described in 1931 (*25*) and again in 1933 it was said to be widespread in the Middle West at that time (*6*). It was seen mostly in hatchery-produced chicks and was thought to be spread from hatcheries. In 1939 the disease was reported as becoming more common and it is now said to be one of the most frequently observed respiratory diseases in Rhode Island (*10*).

Those who investigated the disease were able to reproduce it by inoculation of filtered tracheal exudates from sick birds into the trachea of susceptible birds. The causative agent is now generally regarded as a filterable virus.

Various investigators have reported that chicks were susceptible to the disease as early as the fourth day and as late as the sixth month of age. As in infectious laryngotracheitis, an attack of infectious bronchitis leaves the survivor solidly immune to subsequent exposure to the virus by either natural or artificial means.

It is difficult to make a positive diagnosis distinguishing between infectious bronchitis, infectious laryngotracheitis and infectious coryza, since all three of these respiratory diseases may produce common symptoms and lesions. In a differential diagnosis, the symptoms, lesions, course of the disease, causative agent, morbidity and mortality must all be taken into account. Frequently, cross-immunity tests and bacteriological examination must be made before there can be a positive diagnosis.

The symptoms of bronchitis may include some of those seen in laryngotracheitis and in coryza, such as gasping or mouth breathing, coughing, breathing noises (rales, mucous click), swelling of the nasal sinuses, nasal discharge, watering of the eyes and swelling under the mandible.

The lesions in uncomplicated bronchitis are located in the lungs, whereas in uncomplicated laryngotracheitis the principal tissue changes are found in the larynx and trachea. The lungs are congested and red. The large and small bronchial tubes contain mucopus which later may become cheesy and form solid yellow plugs or casts that exclude the air and produce difficult, gasping breathing. Occasionally unusual cases may be seen in which blood-stained mucopus is present throughout the trachea, as in infectious laryngotracheitis.

The course of the disease has been variously reported to run from 3 or 4 to as many as 8 days, with losses of infected chicks ranging from 10 to over 90 percent.

It has been suggested that the infection may be carried through the egg or by carrier hens, as well as by the excretions of sick birds. It seems probable that the virus may survive in recovered birds for an undetermined period and thus infect younger susceptible chickens.

As in infectious laryngotracheitis, prevention seems to offer the best method of control. On account of the sudden onset and rapid course of the disease in very young chicks, as well as its sporadic nature, preventive vaccination does not seem to be feasible. When attempts are made to immunize chickens against. infectious bronchitis by cloacal vaccination as used for laryngotracheitis, it was found that the virus was carried from the cloaca to the lungs, where the disease developed before immunity could be established as a result of the vaccination.

The disease is spread by infected chicks. Hence, when chicks are purchased they should be carefully inspected for evidence of respiratory infection.

It has been reported that the respiratory distress in young chicks may be ameliorated if it is treated in the early stages by vaporizing the chicks with such volatile oils as menthol, eucalyptol and guaiacol.

After the removal of infected chicks, the brooder house and all utensils should be thoroughly cleaned and disinfected before being restocked with healthy chicks.

It is further recommended that careful attention be paid to heating, ventilation and sanitation in the brooder house, since neglect of these points may predispose the chicks to respiratory disease. The brooder house should be well ventilated without drafts. It should not be allowed to become too hot, dry and dusty. Overcrowding and insanitary conditions are to be avoided.

Infectious Fowl Coryza

Infectious coryza in fowls is an acute inflammatory and contagious disease of the upper air passages. Older names and synonyms are catarrhal roup, cold, rhinitis and sinusitis. Catarrhal diseases of the mucous membranes of the nose, eyes and adjacent sinuses of the fowl were formerly called roup, regardless of the causative agent. Roup, therefore, came to have a very broad meaning, but as the causes of the various catarrhal diseases of the head become known, this term has disappeared from the literature on the subject.

In addition to the nasal passages and adjacent sinuses, the mucous membranes of the eye (conjunctival sac) and the sinuses under the eye frequently become involved.

Beginning in 1932, several investigators reported isolating a bacillus (*Hemophilus gallinarum*) from chickens that were suffering with coryza and reproducing the disease by inoculating the germs into susceptible chickens (*8, 9, 13, 23, 26*). At least two distinct types of coryza are now recognized which are different from a causal as well as a clinical standpoint. The type caused by the germ *H. gallinarum* has a rapid onset and relatively short duration, whereas a second type, the causative agent of which has not been determined with certainty, takes 9 to 27 days to develop and lasts 2 months or longer.

In California two types of coryza have been reported, a mild type with only a nasal discharge and a severe type with complications. In the former, the course was short and the losses were negligible. The most common complication was an edematous swelling of the face, which in males sometimes extended to the wattles. Other complications were inflammation of the sinuses, conjunctivae, trachea and bronchial tubes and air-sac infection.

When the lower respiratory tract was involved there were coughing and gasping. When complications were present the course of the disease was prolonged from several weeks to several months. The mortality varied from a few cases to more than 50 percent of a flock.

A coryza caused by the fowl cholera bacillus, *Pasteurella avicida*, has been reported (*19, 24*). It was found that when fowl cholera has been prevalent in a flock for some time the cholera bacillus loses virulence and tends to become localized in different parts of the body. The reaction to this local infection varies with the individual; some develop sinusitis, or ocular roup, whereas others become healthy carriers. It is thought the latter may cause the annual occurrence of colds among susceptible pullets each year.

When there is only a simple discharge from the nose, coryza is easy to diagnose, but when complications intervene, such as swelling of the face and wattles and gasping or coughing, diagnosis becomes a problem. Coryza must then be differentiated from cholera infection, infectious laryngotrachelitis and infectious bronchitis. A differential diagnosis can be made with certainty only by means of a bacteriological examination and cross-immunity tests, which are carried out as already described for laryngotracheitis.

Infectious coryza begins with a watery exudate from the nose and often from the eyes as well. In a short time the exudate, which usually has a very offensive odour, becomes thick and sticky. As it dries around the nostrils and eyelids, the latter tend to stick together. In some cases exudate accumulates in the nasal sinuses and those under the eyes in large, cheesy masses which exert pressure on the eye, closing it (Fig. 3) and sometimes destroying the sight. There may be a watery (edematous) swelling of the entire face and wattles (Fig. 4).

In an outbreak in Rhode Island, an elevation of body temperature at the onset was reported. The disease spread rapidly, with a high mortality which was ascribed to the presence of some toxic principle. The principal symptoms were a discharge from the nasal passages and sinusitis. There was also considerable involvement of the eyes, with reddening, swelling, watering and sensitiveness to light. The larynx, trachea, or bronchial tube were little affected. Sick birds lost their appetities and rapidly became emaciated. On the other hand, it has also been reported that birds artificially infected by injection of the coryza bacillus did not appear ill and few died, but growth was

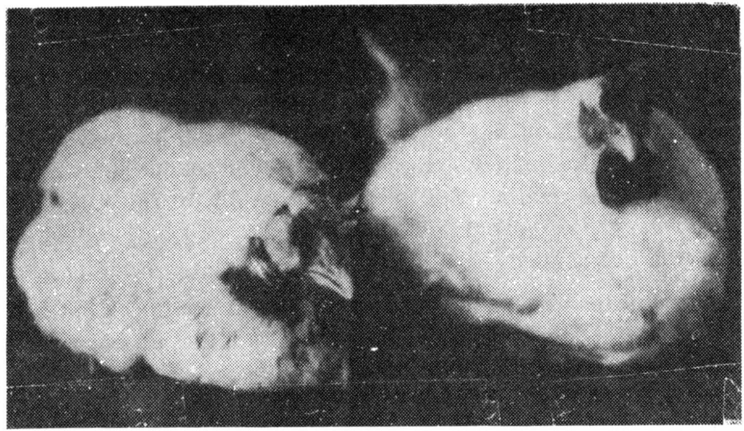

Fig. 3: Results of a natural infection with infectious fowl coryza. Left, severe swelling of the head; right, slight facial swelling and conjunctivitis. (Courtesy of the Division of Veterinary Science, California Agricultural Experiment Station).

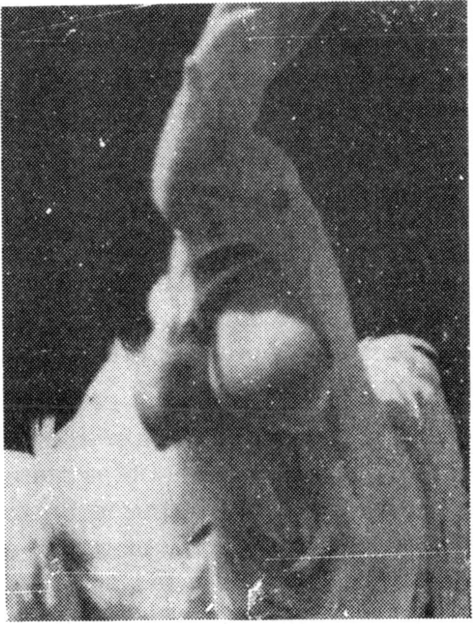

Fig. 4: Swelling of the entire face and wattles produced by injection of a culture of *Hemophilus gallinarum*, the causative agent of infectious fowl coryza, into the wattles. (Courtesy of the Division of Veterinary Science, California Agricultural Experiment Station.)

retarded and egg production was depressed; in about 10 percent of the cases there were secondary manifestations such as tracheal involvement, with noisy breathing and gasping.

Recently it has been found that sulfathiazole administered at the rate of approximately 4 grams per pound of feed, or 1 percent is effective in the treatment of the acute type of coryza caused by *Hemophilus gallinarum* but its effect on other types of coryza has not been fully determined (*10a*).

The means by which the disease is spread from flock to flock under natural conditions are not known. It appears probable that recovered birds may become carriers, as in infectious laryngotracheitis and infectious bronchitis. It has been demonstrated that as long as 46 days after recovery fowls may be carriers of the causative agent of the disease, but that cages and feed and water vessels contaminated by a virulent exudate from infected chickens did not remain infective to susceptible chickens for more than 24 hours. The disease is readily transmitted by placing infected chickens in the same pen with susceptible chickens.

In contrast to the solid, lasting immunity induced by an attack of infectious laryngotracheitis and infectious bronchitis, the immunity of birds that have recovered from an attack of infectious coryza has been reported to be temporary.

It is recommended that careful attention should be paid to housing and to the nutrition of the pullets when they go into the laying house. Drafts, insufficient ventilation, overcrowding, dampness and insanitary conditions should be avoided so as not to lower the natural resistance of the birds.

The yearly occurrence of colds among pullets in California (7) has been attributed to the carrying over of the causative agent by fowls that recovered from an attack during the previous year. Recommendations for control include the complete segregation of pullets from flocks held over from the previous year by (1) depopulation–disposal of all old flocks–and cleaning and disinfecting the quarters occupied by these flocks before bringing in a new stock of pullets; and (2) segregation -the old stock to be removed to houses as far from the pullet quarters as possible so that there is no contact between the two groups.

Non-Infectious Coryzas

Coryzalike symptoms–a nasal discharge and swelling of the sinuses or chalky deposits in the conjunctival sac–may also be caused by vitamin A deficiency, sometimes referred to as nutritional roup, or by mechanical irritation by foreign particles and these conditions may be confused with infectious coryza.

In the non-infectious coryza caused by vitamin A deficiency there is usually a thin, watery discharge from the nostrils, followed by a grayish-white, cheesy deposit in the conjunctival sac and sometimes in the nasal cleft, in the mouth and on the pharynx and gullet, where the deposit occurs as white, pinhead-size nodules. Postmortem examination sometimes reveals white, chalky deposits in the heart sac, on the surface of the liver and in the kidneys.

Nutritional coryza may be cured by increasing the proportion in the diet of vitamin A rich supplements such as green feed, yellow corn, cod-liver oil, alfalfa leaf meal and carrots.

Occasionally sporadic cases of non-infectious coryza may occur as the result of irritation of the mucous membranes of the nasal sinuses and eyelids by foreign particles such as dust, grain, litter and disinfectant chemicals. The irritation may set up inflammation of the mucous membranes, which is followed by a discharge of mucus and pus. This type of non-specific coryza is infrequent. The symptoms may be in distinguishable from those of infectious coryza, but only an occasional bird is affected and the disease does not spread.

Sinusitis (Roup, Swellhead) in Turkeys

A form of coryza in turkeys is characterized by swelling of the sinuses under the eyes. From a causative standpoint two types are described, one infectious and one nutritional, but the causative agent in the so-called infectious type has not yet been found.

The first symptom of the infectious type of the disease is a thin, watery discharge from the nostrils, which soon becomes thick and adhesive. The bird shakes it head and wipes its face on its feathers in an effort to dislodge the discharge. This is followed by bulging or swelling of the face just below and in front of the eye due to the filling of the sinus with an exudate that resembles thin egg albumen. The swelling may appear on one or both sides of the face and in some cases it obstructs vision so that the bird is unable to eat.

In outbreaks in Utah it was found that the swellings varied in size from a slight enlargement to one the size of a hen's egg. It was also reported that sinusitis in turkeys differs from that in chickens in that the exudate consists of a yellowish mucus which remains liquid, whereas in the chicken it becomes cheesy. Only in cases of long standing do the contents of the sinuses in the turkeys become caseous, or cheesy. Although early spontaneous recovery sometimes occurs, the infectious type of the disease usually persists in a flock for weeks or months. The course is more prolonged in those cases in which the exudate becomes firm and cheesy.

In addition to the symptoms and lesions described for the infectious type, the nutritional type, caused by an insufficient amount of vitamin A in the diet, has been reported to show a whitish exudate in the eye in over 80 percent of the cases; pustules in the mouth and esophagus in over 30 percent and in the crop in 60 percent; a catarrhal or cheesy exudate in the bursa of Fabricius in nearly 70 percent; white deposits of urates in the kidneys and body cavities in a few cases; and occasionally a cheesy plug in the larynx or a tubular cast in the trachea.

In all the outbreaks described, losses to the grower were said to be heavy, not so much from mortality as from loss of flesh and unsalability of the birds. In California (*11*) the mortality was low, but the morbidity (percentage of sick birds) was from 10 to 90 percent of the flock. The disease occurs widely in New South Wales (*16*), Australia, where it causes heavy losses and considerable mortality. It occurs most frequently in birds 3 to 5 months of age, but it may also affect birds a few weeks old and among the latter the mortality is said to be heavy.

In making a diagnosis it should be determined whether the disease is of the infectious or nutritional type. The nutritional type of sinusitis may be prevented by providing the birds with a sufficient amount of vitamin A in the diet through the use of green feed, yellow corn, alfalfa leaf meal, or cod-liver oil. It has been shown that turkey poults require nearly twice as much vitamin A rich supplements to maintain health as do chicks (*17*).

A diet containing adequate amounts of vitamin A is also desirable; to build up resistance to the so-called infectious sinusitis. Overcrowding, in sanitary conditions and exposure to drafts and storms should be avoided.

Infectious sinusitis in turkeys can be successfully treated by evacuating the sinus and injecting argyrol or silver nitrate. Some investigators report that silver nitrate is preferable for turkeys and others have reported that a 15 percent solution of fresh argyrol was ineffective when injected into the infraorbital sinuses of fowls affected with coryza (*12*).

The procedure used in California for the treatment of sinusitis in turkeys is as follows: The swollen sinus is emptied by inserting a hypodermic needle of large (*12* or *15*) gage attached to a glass syringe (Luer type) into the lower portion of the sinus and then slowly withdrawing the plunger, thus drawing the mucus into the syringe. Care should be taken not to damage the wall of the sinus or the mucous membrane in inserting the syringe or withdrawing the exudate so as not to clog the needle by sucking in the mucous membrane. After withdrawal of the exudate from the swollen sinus, the syringe may be detached from the needle, which is left in the sinus. Another syringe containing 15 percent fresh argyrol, or 4 percent silver nitrate is attached to the needle and about 1 cubic centimeter is injected into the sinus. The sinus may then be gently massaged before withdrawal of the needle. Care should be observed not to inject the medicine into the tissues surrounding the sinus, as this may cause severe inflammation and sloughing. With this treatment the swelling subsides in 2 or 3 days and in the majority of cases recovery is complete in about 2 weeks. A few cases require a second treatment.

In Utah two techniques have been used. In one, an incision about three-eighths of an inch in length was made over the sinus with a sharp, pointed knife and the exudate was forced out through the incision by massage. Through the opening 15 to 20 drops of medicinal solution (20 percent arurol or 4 percent silver nitrate) was instilled by means of a medicine dropper. In cases where bleeding was severe the sinus was packed with cotton, In the other technique, a 10 to 20 cubic centimeter hypodermic syringe, fitted with a 16 gage needle 1½ inches long, was used to empty the sinus. Another syringe fitted with a smaller needle (18 gage) was used to inject 1 cubic centimeter of the medicine into the sinus, through the hole made by the larger needle. The syringe technique was preferred to the knife technique (22).

Good results were obtained in Australia in the treatment of sinusitis in turkeys by the use of 2 to 5 percent silver nitrate. It is said that new cases respond best to treatment, whereas long-standing cases in which the sinus contents are cheeselike are refractory.

In still another treatment technique the contents of the sinus were evacuated through the orifice leading into the nasal cavity by gentle massage of the swollen sinus, after which 1 to 2 cubic centimeters of fresh 15 percent argyrol was injected (*28*).

An attack of the disease is said to confer immunity to a second attack, but successful immunization of turkeys by subcutaneous injection of the exudate or by application of the exudate to the mucous membrane of the cloaca has not been reported.

Literature Cited

(1) BEACH, J.R. (1930). THE VIRUS OF LARYNGOTRACHEITIS OF FOWLS. Science 72; 633-634.

(2) _____(1931). A BACTERIOLOGICAL STUDY OF INFECTIOUS LARYNGOTRACHEITIS OF CHICKENS; Jour. Expt. Med. 54: 801-808.

(3) BEAUDETTE, F.R. (1930). BRONCHITIS IN POULTRY. N.J. Agr. 12 (5): 3, 4.

(4) _____and HUDSON, C.B. (1933). EXPERIMENTS ON IMMUNIZATION AGAINST LARYNGOTRACHEITIS IN FOWLS. Amer. Vet. Med. Assoc. Jour. 82: 460-476.

(5) BRANDLY, C.A. (1934). SOME STUDIES OF INFECTIOUS LARYNGOTRACHEITIS. Amer. Vet. Med. Assoc. Jour. 84: 588-595.

(6) BUSHNELL, L.D. and BRANDLY, C.A. (1933). LARYNGOTRACHEITIS IN CHICKS. Poultry Sci. 12: 55-60.

(7) BUSIC, W.H. and BEACH, J.R. (1934). HANDLING COLDS ON POULTRY FARMS. Pacific Rural Press 128: 368.

(8) DE-BLIECK, L. (1932). A HAEMOGLOBINOPHILIC BACTERIUM AS THE CAUSE OF CONTAGIOUS CATARRH OF THE FOWL. (CORYZA INFECTIOSA GALLINARUM). Vet. Jour. 88: 9-13.

(9) DELAPLANE, J.P., ERWIN, L.E. and STUART, H.O. (1934). A HEMOPHILIC BACILLUS AS THE CAUSE OF AN INFECTIOUS RHINITIS. R.I. Agr. Expt. Sta. Bull. 244, 12 pp., illus.

(10) _____and STUART, H.O. (1939). STUDIES OF INFECTIOUS BRONCHITIS. R.I. Expt. Sta. Bull. 273, 15 pp.

(10a)_____and STUART, H.O. (1941). THE CHEMOTHERAPEUTIC VALUE OF SULFATHIAZOLE IN PREVENTING AND TREATING INFECTIOUS

CORYZA (HEMOPHILUS GALLINARUM INFECTION) IN CHICKENS. Am. Vet. Med. Assoc. Jour. 99 (772): 41-42.

(11) DICKINSON, E.M. and HINSHAW, W.R. (1938). TREATMENT OF INFECTIOUS SINUSITIS OF TURKEYS WITH ARGYROL AND SILVER NITRATE. Amer. Vet. Med. Assoc. Jour. 93: 151-156, illus.

(12) _____and BEACH, J.R. (1938). TREATMENT OF FOWL CORYZA OF CHICKENS WITH ARGYROL. Amer. Vet. Med. Assoc: Jour. 93: 108.

(13) ELIOT, CALISTA P. and LEWIS, MARGARET, R. (1934). A HEMOPHILIC BACTERIUM AS A CAUSE OF INFECTIOUS CORYZA IN THE FOWL. Amer. Vet. Mcd. Assoc. Jour. 84: 878-888.

(14) GIBBS, CHARLES S. (1931). INFECTIOUS TRACHITIS. Mass. Agr. Expt. Sta. Bull. 273, pp. [25]-55, illus.

(15) GRAHAM, ROBERT, THORP, FRANK. JR. and JAMES, W.A. (1931). A FILTERABLE VIRUS-LIKE AGENT IN AVIAN LARYNGOTRACHEITIS. Amer. Vet. Med. Assoc. Jour. 78: 506.

(16) HART, L. (1940). SINUSITIS IN TURKEYS. Austral. Vet. Jour. 16: 163-168, illus.

(17) HINSHAW, W.R. and LLOYD, W.E. (1934). VITAMIN-A DEFICIENCY IN TURKEYS. Hilgardia 8: 281-304, illus.

(18) HUDSON, C.B. and BEAUDETTE, F.R. (1932). INFECTION OF THE CLOACA WITH THE VIRUS OF INFECTIOUS BRONCHITIS. Science 76; 34.

(19) HUGHES, THOMAS P. and PRITCHETT, IDA W. (1930). THE EPIDEMIOLOGY OF FOWL CHOLERA. III. PORTAL OF ENTRY OF P. AVIOIDA; REACTION OF THE HOST. Jour. Expt. Med. 51: 239-248, illus.

(20) HUNGERFORD, T.G. (1938). INFECTIOUS LARYNGOTRAOHEITIS. Agr. Gaz. N. S. Wales 49: 628-632, illus.

(21) KERNOHAN, GEORGE (1931). INFEOTIOUS LARYNGOTRACHEITIS OF FOWLS. Amer. Vet. Med. Assoc. Jour. 78: 196-202.

(22) MADSEN, D.E. (1938). SINUSITIS OF TURKEYS. Utah Agr. Expt. Sta. Bull. 280, 12 pp., illus.

(23) NELSON, JOHN B. (1932). ETIOLOGY OF AN UNCOMPLICATED CORYZA IN THE DOMESTIC FOWL. Soc. Exp. Biol. and Med. Proc. 30: 306-307.

(24) PRITCHETT, IDA W., BEAUDEITE, F.R. and HUGHES, T.P. (1930). THE EPIDEMIOLOGY OF FOWL CHOLERA. IV. FIELD OBSERVATIONS OF THE "SPONTANEOUS" DISEASE. Jour. Expt. Med. 51: 249-258.

(25) SOHALK, A.F. and HAWN, M.C. (1931). AN APPARENTLY NEW RESPIRATORY DISEASE OF BABY CHICKS. Amer. Vet. Med. Assoc. Jour. 78: 413-422.

(26) SCHALM, O.W. and BFACH, J.R. (1934). THE ETIOLOGY OF A RESPIRATORY DISEASE OF CHICKENS. Science 79: 416-417.

(27) _____and BEACH, J.R. (1935). THE RESISTANCE OF THE VIRUS OF INFECTIOUS LARYNGOTRACHEITIS TO CERTAIN PHYSICAL AND CHEMICAL FACTORS. Jour. Infect. Dis. 56: [210]-223.

(28) TYZZER, E.E. (1926). THE INJECTION OF ARGYROL FOR THE TBEATMENT OF SINUSITIS.IN TURKEYS. Cornell Vet. 16: 221-224.

Chapter 4

FOWL POX (DIPHTHERIA)

Hubert Bunyea [1]

[1] *Hubert Bunyea is Veterinarian, Pathological Division, Bureau of Animal Industry.*

The skin form of fowl pox is a comparatively mild disease, but it has a diphtheritic form that can be extremely serious. Fortunately, it is one of the diseases for which successful vaccination methods have been developed.

Fowl Pox is a disease complex consisting of lesions, or tissue injuries, of the skin (pox) and of the mucous membranes (diphtheria). It affects many species of domestic fowls and free-flying wild birds.

It is now known that fowl pox is caused by an invisible disease producing agency. From time to time many agents, including bacteria and protozoa of various kinds, have been believed to produce the disease. In an old book on poultry diseases[2] the origin of diphtheria is attributed mainly to "improper care and sudden changes of weather and variations of temperature," and the author adds that "it is also occasioned by improper and damp coops and roosts." About the beginning of the present century, however, it was discovered that infectious material from pox-infected fowls was capable of retaining its disease-producing power even after it had

---

[2] LEWIS, W.M. THE PEOPLE'S PRACTICAL POULTRY BOOK. Ed. 7, 223 pp., illus. New York. 1876.

passed through filters too fine to permit the passage of bacteria. Such an infective agent is known as a filtrable virus.

Two types or strains of the virus are known to be infectious for avian species. The more common and more important strain causes natural outbreaks in chickens and other barnyard fowl, including turkeys, guinea fowl, pheasants, ducks, geese and other species. Of less importance is pigeon pox virus, which as its name implies, produces the disease in pigeons. Other species are relatively resistant to pigeon pox virus, but it has produced mild lesions experimentally in chickens, particularly when inoculated into feather follicles, a fact that is the basis for immunization of chickens with this type of the virus, as discussed later. Pigeons are quite resistant to the other type.

The virus of fowl pox, or chicken pox, is very resistant to desiccation, or drying. Infectious matter from the diseased birds may therefore be scattered around the premises and will remain in a dried condition for many months, during which time it may come into contact with susceptible birds and bring about a new outbreak. Such an outbreak usually begins with the occurrence of the typical pox lesions on the face parts of the fowls. The virus may gain entrance where the comb or wattle has been wounded, possibly during fights with other birds. Certain species of mosquitoes may spread the disease by carrying the infection from a diseased fowl to a susceptible one. A mosquito may be infectious for as long as 27 days after feeding on an infected fowl.

It is probable that the disease is transmitted only through damaged or broken skin or mucous membranes. Wounds too small to be observed may afford an entrance for the virus into the skin.

Fowl pox virus is not infectious for human beings or any species of mammal; so-called chicken pox (varicella) in human beings is an entirely distinct disease. Fowls and free-flying birds of any age are susceptible to fowl pox. Usually, however, very young and very old birds are not affected, probably because the young birds are more sheltered from exposure and the old birds have in many cases survived a previous outbreak and developed immunity. Fowls of any breed and practically all species are susceptible to the disease; Large-combed and large-wattled birds seem to acquire the pox lesions more often, probably because the greater surface of these parts exposed to skin wounds. The diphtheria manifestations affect all breeds equally.

Symptoms

The cutaneous (pox) lesions are usually the first to appear, the membranous (diphtheria) lesions occurring later. The infection gains a foothold in the flock through the pox lesions, but in the diphtheritic form it may persist longer and do greater damage. Fowl pox may appear at any season, though as a rule it is more likely to occur in the fall or winter.

The pox manifestations, known as fowl pox, bird pox, chicken pox, sorehead, dry pox, avian molluscum, or contagious epithelioma, occur as wartlike nodules (Fig. 1) on the unfeathered parts of the body such as the comb, wattles, eyelids and vent. The diphtheritic manifestations, known as avian diphtheria, diphtheritic roup, wet pox or canker, occur as a deposit on the mucous membranes of the eyes, mouth, or respiratory region and are sometimes accompanied by coughing and gasping. Both types of lesion frequently occur in a single outbreak of the disease.

For many years the two manifestations were regarded as entirely distinct diseases due to different infective agents. Within comparatively recent times, however, it has been clearly demonstrated that the two disease manifestations have a common origin. Virus collected from pox lesions has been shown by inoculation to be infective for the membranes of the eye, mouth and air passages, whereas virus collected from diphtheria lesions, when rubbed into scarified (scraped) areas on the comb, wattles, or other parts of a fowl's body, has been shown to be capable of producing typical pox lesions.

In the cutaneous, or pox, manifestation of the infection, the lesions appear 3 to 4 days after exposure, in the form of minute grayish pimples or blisters, usually on the unfeathered parts of the fowl's body. The blisters contain a straw-coloured fluid which is very virulent. In the course of several days they begin to enlarge and run together. Meanwhile the skin around the blisters takes on an angry, red appearance. After 10 to 14 days, the blisters may begin to darken and form day, hard scabs resembling warts, which may cling to the skin for another week or two or even longer. Finally the scabs loosen and drop off, revealing new and possible scarred skin beneath.

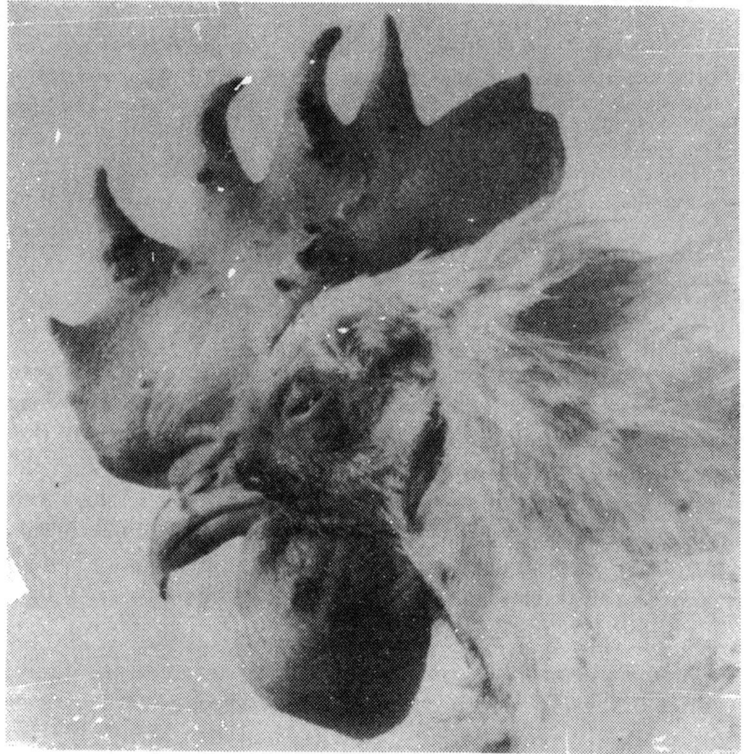

Fig. 1: Pox lesions on comb, wattle, eyelid, and mouth parts of a chicken.

In the diptheritic form the disease has no definite course, but may persist for weeks or possibly months before it is terminated by death or recovery. Yellowish or whitish chessy patches form on the mucous membrane of the tongue, mouth, esophagus and larynx. The patches of membrane like material found in some cases within the trachea may cause gaping and laboured breathing, which may be mistaken for symptoms of infectious laryngotracheitis. The patches are very tough and adherent. If forcibly removed, they, leave the true membrane in a bleeding and ulcerous condition. Similar deposits may occur in the sinuses of the eye, preceded by watering and inflammation. The eyelids eventually become swollen and tend to stick together. This type of diphtheria is sometimes incorrectly alluded to as diphtheritic roup.

The presence of the cheesy membranous deposits in the mouth, eyes and air passages interferes seriously with the bird's vision and respiration and tends to interfere with its eating. As a result, progressive emaciation sets in and egg production definitely and sometimes permanently stops. Weakness, starvation and in many cases suffocation precede death. Recovery may occur in mild cases of diphtheria, imparting prolonged immunity, as does recovery from the cutaneous or pox manifestations of the disease.

Mortality and Economic Importance

The cutaneous pox manifestations are usually mild and after a fairly definite period terminate in an uneventful recovery. The diphtheritic type of infection, however, may cause more or less mortality among the birds, the rate being influenced by the age of the birds and general health conditions in the flock. Other things being equal, the death rate is highest among pullets in egg production. However, complication with other diseases of a debilitating nature, poor nutrition, bad housing conditions, severe weather, or even a moderately heavy parasitic infestation will increase the losses.

No authentic statistics on the economic loss to the poultry industry occasioned by this disease are available. It has been estimated that uncontrolled outbreaks may cost poultry keepers $30 to $70 per hundred birds. Losses are chargeable to such items, in addition to mortality, as the time, work and equipment used in isolating and treating sick birds; the loss of vitality of sick birds; the suppression of egg production in affected birds–many do not return to production for a number of months and some never regain normal production; the decreased reproductive power in breeding stock; and the predisposition of affected birds to other diseases.

Treatment and Control

In severe outbreaks medicinal treatment is usually of little or no value. Birds lightly affected, if of more than ordinary value, may be removed from the flock and placed under quarantine in comfortable quarters. The false membrane should be removed from the mouth or larynx so that the bird may eat and breathe more easily. Tincture of iodine, argyrol, or iodoform powder should be applied to the underlying ulcers to promote healing. The drinking water should be made antiseptic by the addition of one-third of a dram (one-third teaspoonful) of potassium permanganate crystals per gallon. Strict sanitation should be observed in the quarantine house and the attendant, if possible, should refrain from visiting the quarters of the healthy flock. Changing clothes and disinfecting the footwear should be done faithfully after working in the quarantine house.

No special control measures can be recommended for fowl pox. General hygienic precautions should be adopted. Affected birds should be segregated and, if in a serious condition, may as well be slaughtered since the likelihood of their becoming profitable is remote. The premises from which sick birds have been removed for quarantine or slaughter should be thoroughly cleansed and disinfected. A good disinfectant for this purpose may be made by dissolving 1 pound of commercial lye (containing 94 percent of sodium hydroxide) and 2½ pounds of water-slaked lime in 5½ gallons of water. Unless kept tightly covered, this solution will deteriorate on standing. It is injurious to painted or varnished surfaces, aluminium utensils and some fabrics, but it is relatively harmless to the equipment usually found around chicken houses.

Precautions should be taken against introducing the disease in pox-free flocks or areas. So far as possible, wild birds should be excluded from contact with the flock and prevented from visiting premises used for poultry. Visitors who own poultry that may be harbouring the infection should not be permitted access to the flock, or, if this is unavoidable, they should be provided with a pair of clean rubbers. Hucksters, peddlers, feed dealers and other itinerant persons are potential transmitters of infection, as they frequently visit many poultry establishments in a day and they should by all means be excluded from the poultry houses. Veterinarians and officials engaged in various lines of poultry work may be expected to take what precautions are necessary to avoid transmitting infections from place to place in the discharge of their duties.

Vaccination

If the outbreak is light and of recent origin, vaccination of the healthy birds may be resorted to after removal of the affected ones. After the disease has been present for several weeks or months, however, vaccination is of doubtful value. Birds that remain healthy for that long may be presumed to be resistant; it is always possible that they may have acquired unseen pox lesions and have thereby developed immunity. The fact that fowls that recover from the disease possess a solid immunity to further attack for a considerable length of time has been the basis for much of the experimental work that has led to the present methods of vaccination of poultry for the prevention of fowl pox.

As early as 1910, investigators reported favourable results from the injection into the veins of pox-scab material ground in a physiological, salt solution (one that is like the body fluids). Later workers announced the production of immunity in fowls injected twice at 5 day intervals with a saline suspension of pox scabs and diphtheritic membrane that had been filtered and heated for an hour at 55° C (131° F.). These methods, however, failed to gain wide acceptance owing to the lack of uniformly satisfactory results.

Within the last 22 years a definitely successful procedure has been developed for the immunization of chickens against pox. The basic agent employed is the living virus of chicken pox or of pigeon pox. Instead of these materials being injected under the skin or into the veins, they are applied by superficial, stabs into the skin or to four or six follicles from which the feathers have been plucked. Except in the stab, or stick, method the vaccine is usually vigorously applied with a bristle brush to the prepared area. A successful vaccination is followed by the development of a typical pox lesion at the point of vaccination. Pigeon pox vaccine is applied only to the feather follicles; 12 to 20 feathers are plucked and the follicles are inoculated (Fig. 2). In employing the stab method, any clean, sterile, sharp-pointed instrument may be used that will penetrate the skin and convey a minute amount of the virus to the inoculated area. A popular method is to bind two sewing-machine needles to the end of a wooden handle about the thickness of a lead pencil, leaving exposed only the eyes of the needles. When this instrument, after being disinfected, is dipped into the vaccine suspension, sufficient vaccine is picked-up in the eyes of the needles to inoculate the skin on both sides of the wing. The needles are then thrust through the web of one wing. This method is economical, efficient and speedy. Other parts of the skin, such as the thigh, may be inoculated if preferred.

The vaccine is a standardized powder consisting of material that came originally from pox scabs, thoroughly dried and finely pulverized. Under proper conditions, the powder will retain its potency for a long time. For immediate use it is usually mixed with a sterilized fluid consisting of equal parts of glycerine and physiological salt solution. This fluid suspension of the vaccine is

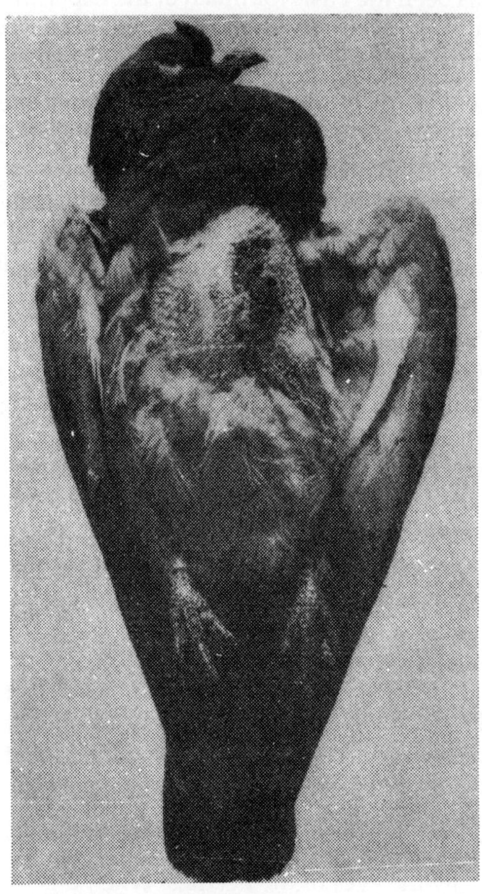

Fig. 2: Pigeon pox vaccination lesion on the breast of a pigeon.

very short-lived. It should be kept from exposure to extreme temperatures, excessive sunlight, or atmospheric contamination and any part remaining unused at the end of the day should be destroyed by burning or disinfection.

Within the last decade it has been discovered that certain viruses, including those of fowl pox and pigeon pox, can be propagated on the embryonic tissue in incubated eggs of chickens. This method of propagation, which eliminates the necessity of constantly collecting virus from actual cases, has therefore come into use for the production of virus vaccines. It is more economical than methods previously employed for preparing fowl pox and pigeon pox vaccines, and, when properly produced, such vaccine has been found to be as potent as that made from pox scabs.

The question is sometimes asked, "if a natural outbreak of fowl pox will produce immunity, why go to the bother of vaccinating?" The reasons may be summed up about as follows:

1. To prevent the possible losses that might result if the disease were allowed to run its course. Vaccination is likely to be considerably cheaper than natural immunity.
2. To speed up the production of immunity.
3. To have some control over the time of occurrence of the disease (vaccination is an artificial production of the disease). Without vaccination, a natural outbreak might occur at a most inconvenient time and might take a long time to go through a flock.
4. To be sure that the lesions have time to heal completely before egg production begins. (Vaccination as well as a natural outbreak immediately prior to or during egg production is likely to depress productivity.)
5. To control the size and location of the lesions. Occasionally the disease spreads from the vaccinated area to other parts of the body and it may even break out in the diphtheritic form. As a rule, however, the lesion remains confined to the vaccinated area and does not appreciably enlarge.

Birds that have been vaccinated within a year with fowl pox vaccine or that have recovered from the disease within that period may be presumed to be immune. Pigeon pox vaccine imparts only temporary immunity of a relatively low degree. Birds previously vaccinated with the pigeon pox vaccine only and all susceptible adults, yearlings, or pullets should be vaccinated with fowl pox vaccine. Baby Chicks should be safeguarded from all contact with the, disease, as it is not considered profitable to attempt to immunize them. Other species on the premises, especially turkeys, guineas and pheasants, should be vaccinated.

The programme of vaccination should not be unduly prolonged but should be completed as rapidly as is compatible with efficient work.

If the work is carried over several days, freshly mixed vaccine should be used each day and birds not yet vaccinated should be kept completely isolated for their own protection. If any adult birds cannot be included, they too must be completely isolated from any contact with the vaccinated birds or their attendants. When pigeon pox vaccine is used, there is little or no danger of the disease spreading among chickens.

Birds to be shipped or to be entered in egglaying contests or exhibitions may be vaccinated with pigeon pox vaccine in order to impart a temporary immunity without undue disturbance of productivity. This vaccine may also be safely employed in protecting a flock approaching the laying season or when the disease has broken out during a period of egg production. Following the cessation of production, however, it would be well to revaccinate the birds with fowl pox vaccine in order to insure a prolonged immunity.

Birds that are weakened by a heavy parasitic infestation or the effects of some other disease condition should not be subjected to vaccination with fowl pox vaccine. Poorly feathered, under-nourished, undersized birds or crowded or otherwise poorly housed flocks are not fit subjects for vaccination.

In areas where it is known that the disease does not exist, vaccination is not necessary or desirable. In the first place, the fowls are in no danger of acquiring the disease, and, secondly, the vaccine itself, being the active principle of the disease, may introduce it into the flock and necessitate a continuous vaccination programme.

Vaccination at various ages and various times of the year has been recommended. It is possible to vaccinate baby chicks, but it has been shown that this temporarily interferes with gains in weight and complications with pullorum disease, coccidiosis and other infections are likely to cause a high mortality from vaccination in young birds.

The practice usually recommended is to vaccinate the pullets with fowl pox vaccine, well before the expected onset of egg production. If possible, vaccination should be performed at least 2 months in advance to permit the flock to recuperate fully from the artificially induced disease before beginning to lay. Vaccination between the ages of 12 to 16 weeks usually allows for such an interval.

Contest or exhibition birds should be immunized in time to recover fully before leaving the premises.

Although pigeon pox vaccine may be used without any appreciable disturbance of the bird's health or productivity, it has the disadvantage, as already noted, of giving only temporary and sometimes partial immunity.

Immunity established with fowl pox vaccine, on the other hand, may endure for 1 or 2 years or even for the life of the bird. The lesions caused by this type of vaccination however, are likely to be severe and may spread to other parts of the body. They usually appear 4 to 9 days after vaccination. Failure of lesions to appear may indicate that the vaccine is impotent or that the bird is already immune. Egg production may be indefinitely postponed by vaccination, or, if it has started, it may be stopped abruptly. The vaccinated birds may be droopy and depressed for a number of days or weeks. Appetite is likely to be impaired. Heavily parasitized or debilitated birds will succumb. Should the artificially induced disease break over into the diphtheritic form, more or less mortality and chronic diphtheria will probably result. However, in the vast majority of flocks, vaccination is not accompanied by these serious after effects and immunity is established in an interval of 2 to 4 weeks.

Practical Suggestions for Vaccination

It is desirable to have one or more assistants in catching and handling the fowls that are to be vaccinated. Adequate help and properly coordinated teamwork play a large part in expediting the work.

In follicular vaccination, the operator plucks from the thigh of the bird the necessary number of feathers (Fig. 3). The same leg or wing should always be vaccinated to facilitate the checking of takes (positive vaccination reactions) later. The flock should be examined for takes in 7 to 10 days. A take is indicated by a typical pox vaccination lesion at the site of inoculation. Birds showing no take should be revaccinated at once with fresh vaccine. A predominating number of no takes suggests either that the flock possesses a certain amount of immunity or that the vaccine used was low or lacking in potency. A history of convalescence from a previous out break of fowl pox would go far to explain the occurrence of no takes following vaccination.

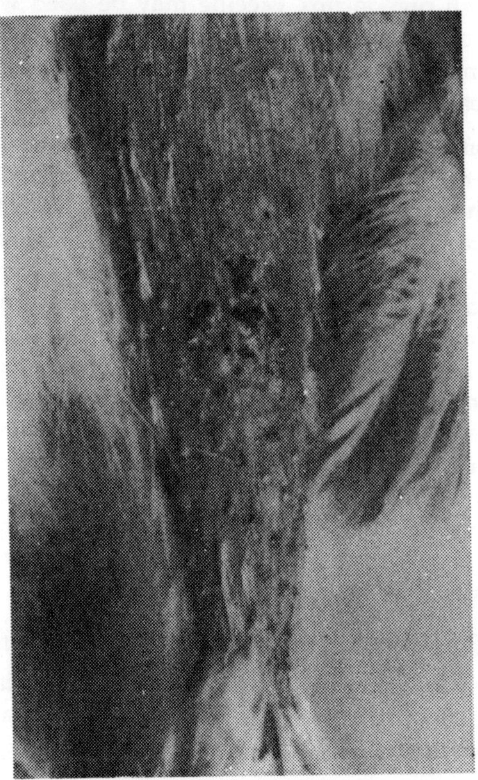

Fig. 3: Follicular vaccination on the thigh of a chicken, showing inoculated and uninoculated (denuded) follicles.

The powdered vaccine should be mixed with the fluid furnished in the package and nothing else. Under no circumstances should additional water or other fluids be added in order to make it go farther or for any other reason. During operations the mixture should be kept from the rays of the sun and from intense heat or freezing and it should be kept covered when not in use, to prevent contamination. It should be used the same day it is mixed. If operations are to be interrupted or suspended for as long as 1 hours or more, the mixed vaccine should be placed in a refrigerator. It should not be used the day after it has been mixed.

In large establishments the work of vaccination may require several days and vaccinated birds should be kept separate from those not yet vaccinated. Systematic procedure will insure that all birds come up for vaccination and that susceptible birds do not come in contact with those that have been vaccinated.

Vaccinated birds are sick birds. They should be made as comfortable as possible, kept dry and be properly fed and watered.

Some operators prefer to vaccinate at night when the fowls are on the roosts. They are quiet then and may be handled with a minimum of disturbance. Adequate illumination must be provided for night vaccination, but the roosts must be shielded from the light in order not to disturb the rest of the flock.

Chapter 5
PSITTACOSIS

K.F. Meyer[1]

[1] *K.F. Meyer is Director of the Hooper Foundation, University of California, San Francisco.*

Psittacosis, a virus disease spread by birds of the parrot family, causes an insidious ailment in human beings that is often hard to distinguish from influenza or pneumonia. Various restrictive measures against birds of the parrot family have been applied in this country in an effort to reduce or wipe out the disease. Recent research discloses the startling fact that the virus may be harboured by other birds, entirely unrelated to parrots–including pigeons and chickens.

It is generally believed that psittacosis is primarily a disease of parrots, parrakeets, or other birds of the parrot family (psittacine birds) which occasionally spread their infection to other cage birds, such as canaries and finches. That these avian maladies may cause serious pneumonias, not typical of ordinary pneumonia, in human beings is well known. It was recognized in 1931[2] that the breeding establishments and aviaries for the raising of parrakeets (*Melopsittacus undulatus* (Shaw) in California harboured apparently healthy birds that were spreading the disease through their droppings. In fact, it was soon realized not only that imported

---

[2] MEYER, K.F., AND EDDIE, B. LATENT PSITTACOSIS INFECTIONS IN SHELL PARRAKEETS. Soc. Expt. Biol. And Med. Proc. 30: 484-488, 1933.

psittacine birds from South America and Australia may be dangerous pets but that the local breeders in the West and in Florida, Texas and even Canada are the disseminators of sickness.

Until a few months ago, however, it was not suspected that barn-yards and pigeon lofts may be sheltering bearers of disease and even death. The unexpected discovery that the disease can exist in such places puts psittacosis in the ranks of diseases of interest and importance to the poultry farmer. Although the available facts are as yet meager, they clearly indicate the magnitude of the problem and the complexity of the control measures that may ultimately required to prevent serious losses and to protect man from this menace.

With the discovery by Haagen and Mauer[3] that psittacosis affects the Arctic fulmar (*Fulmarus glacialis glacialis* L.), or petrel, on the Faroe Islands and the proved susceptibility of the domestic fowl to the germ,[4] it was anticipated that sooner or later infections of other avian species might be encountered. This has happened; but before the observations are recorded it may be advisable to outline briefly the facts about psittacosis known by the end of 1940.

The Human Disease

The term "psittacosis," from the Greek word for parrot, was suggested in 1895 by Morange to designate a peculiar contagious disease of man which had been noted among members of households exposed to sick birds from foreign countries, primarily parrots. In view of the later findings, described in this article, that the disease is more widespread among birds than was at first realized, the name "ornithosis" might be a suitable designation.

The malady became known through localized outbreaks of severe pneumonia in Switzerland in 1879 and in Paris in 1892. These epidemics stopped after a series of orders prohibiting importations of parrots had been issued. Occasionally single or

---

3 HAAGEN, E., AND MAUER, G. UEBEER EINE AUF DEN MENSCHEN UBERTRAGBARE VIRUS KRANKHEIT DIE STURMVOGENLN UND BEZIEHNING ZUR PSITTAKOSE. Nentbl. F.Bakt. (etc.). Originale (I) 143: 81-88, 1938.

4 MEYER, K.F. PSITTACOSIS. 12th Internatl. Vet. Cong. Proc. 3: 182-205, illus. 1935.

group infections were reported from England and the United States, but generally the disease ranked as a medical curiosity. From being a rare and obscure infection, psittacosis became a malady of world-wide interest in 1929-30, when shipments of sick parrots imported from South America into Europe and the United States caused disease in 750 to 800 human beings. The subsequent endemic distribution of psittacosis of parrakeets in the United States, Canada and Germany, which was responsible for an additional 600 recorded human cases, has offered an opportunity to many investigators for a thorough study of the avian as well as the human disease, from the standpoint of its cause as well as its epidemic spread.

It is now firmly established that psittacosis is an infection caused by a filterable bacterium, known as *Microbacterium multiforme psittacosis*, consisting of a protoplasmic cell which can be microscopically demonstrated and cultivated. The hypothesis originally advanced by Nocard that the disease is a *Salmonella* infection has been entirely abandoned.

Household outbreaks follow a typical pattern. An unusual type of pneumonia suddenly develops in a member of a family into which a parrot or a pair of parrakeets, more rarely canaries or finches, have recently been introduced as cage pets. In rapid succession, additional cases occur.among the relatives and even guests or visitors. The responsible birds mayor may not be visibly sick. Usually people of middle age are quite susceptible, whereas children rarely contract the malady.

Human beings suffering from psittacosis or ornithosis complain suddenly of general malaise, chills, headache, restlessness, insomnia, nosebleed and a non-productive cough (without phlegm). The temperature rises rapidly and after a period of continued elevation begins to fall during the second week. As a rule the signs of a peculiar pneumonia appear early in the X-ray picture but it is difficult to distinguish the changes in the lung tissues from those observed in typical influenza. Despite the inflammation in the lung the breathing rate is only slightly increased, usually no chest pain is noted and the number of white blood corpuscles does not increase as in typical pneumonia. The patient is unable to raise much sputum. Since these signs are not distinct enough for diagnosis, an examination of the sputum and a blood test are the diagnostic aids commonly used. Convalescence is slow and tedious. The mortality rate, given as 20 percent, is probably too high, since mild, unreported cases are undoubtedly frequent. The younger the individual the greater is the likelihood that the infection will be mild and a typical-like grippe. There is no specific treatment, though serum from recovered patients may reduce the mortality rate.

Occupational liability among persons engaged in the breeding and trading of psittacine birds is high. Labouratory workers, physicians and sanitary inspectors also frequently contract the disease during the execution of their professional duties. Furthermore, it is important to emphasize that the sputum of patients is sometimes highly infectious and thus transmission from one human being to another is by no means infrequent.

The infection may be passed from bird to man in one of two ways: (1) Inhalation of dust contaminated with infective particles from dried fecal droppings, urine, feathers, ere. and droplets from the nasal secretions of sick or healthy birds, or (2) by direct contact through bites, though this is rare. The high infectivity of the psittacosis virus, which resembles that of smallpox or measles, is, reflected in the histories in which fleeting exposure occurred in a pet shop where diseased birds had been kept. Since air currents may disseminate the virus, actual contact with diseased psittacine birds is not necessary.

Without any definite history of exposure to tropical birds or parrakeets, it is difficult to differentiate psittacosis from influenza or some of the virus pneumonias without labouratory aid. The sputum, if it is raised by the patient in sufficient amounts, may be tested by injecting a suspension of the excretion into the peritoneum, or lining of the abdominal cavity, of white mice. These rodents are extremely susceptible to psittacosis and usually succumb to the infection in 5 to 14 days. In recent years the blood test (complement-fixation test) with specially prepared reagents has proved of great value in the early diagnosis of human infections; moreover, it is useful in discovering the existence of psittacosis in aviaries.

The Disease in Tropical Birds and Finches

The recognition that avian psittacosis of undetermined origin but as a natural disease is common among the cockatoos, lorikeets, cockateels and rosellas of the Australian bush, probably serving as a population regulator and the discovery that shell parrakeets bred and raised in the United States, Canada and Europe and parrots from Panama and Mexico may act as sources of infection are important contributions resulting from the researches conducted since 1931. Particularly far reaching, however, is the finding that apparently healthy birds may harbour the virus and disseminate it. The incidence of these unrecognized latent infections in aviaries and breeding establishments may range from 10 to 90 percent.

With the aid of the so-called mouse-inoculation test or the blood-serum test, it is now practical to detect these carriers. The suspected large birds are bled from the wing vein; the smaller birds are killed, portions of the liver, spleen and kidneys carefully ground up and suspensions of the organs inoculated into white mice or Java rice-birds. When the psittacosis virus is present in the tissues of the suspected birds, the experimental animals acquire the infection and frequently die, providing significant autopsy and microscopic findings. It is important to remember that the clinical manifestations of psittacosis in parrots, parrakeets, canaries, or finches are by no means characteristic and without labouratory tests the identity of the illness cannot be determined.

In many of the importations, the mortality among the parrots has been very high, whereas in the breeding establishments housing parrakeets under fairly sanitary conditions rarely more than 5 to 10 percent succumb to acute psittacosis. It is well known, however, that many of the pen mates of sick birds carry the infective agent, and when brought under adverse environmental conditions, such as crowding, malnutrition and lack of sunlight, these chronically infected birds may suffer relapses. At autopsy, emaciation, an enlarged saffron-coloured liver studded with wedge-shaped pale areas of destroyed tissue (infarcts) and a spleen tumor are usually observed. Preparations made from the tissues reveal colonies and clusters of the elementry bodies in large numbers.

Young birds are more susceptible than older ones; the young ones contract the infection in the nests and whether they are visibly sick, or not they may spread the infection for many months and thus maintain the disease indefinitely in breeding establishments or pet shops. The virus-carrying excreta may soil the food and water; hence it is not surprising that contaminated birdseed from pet shops may occasionally cause new infections in cage birds not directly exposed to diseased parrakeets or parrots.

Public health officials are principally concerned with the elimination of infected psittacine birds from the retail trade in pet shops. Some degree of protection has been obtained by such restrictive measures as an embargo on imported birds, quarantines for not less than 6 months and isolation. The recent outbreaks of Psittacosis in, zoological gardens, however, amply attest to the inadequacy of these precautionary measures. Certain States, including Connecticut, New York and Oregon, maintain a permanent quarantine against psittacine birds.

Since the commercial aviaries engaged in the breeding and raising of shell parrakeets are the principal distributors of diseased birds and the sources of severe outbreaks (epizootics) among canaries and finches in pet shops, California has attempted to free the bird industry from Psittacosis in that State. Anyone engaged in selling, trading, or bartering shell parrakeets must obtain a certificate of registration (California Senate Bill 516, 1933). According to regulations, the aviaries must furnish 10 to 20 percent of the birds for two labouratory tests before they may be certified and the birds released for sale. The parrakeets are killed and their viscera tested for virus through inoculation of mice. Aviaries, found to harbour birds with the psittacosis virus are quarantined and the owners are advised to destroy their stocks. The birds of a certified aviary wear a leg band with a code number assigned to them by the California State Department of Public Health. For interstate shipment, the United States Public Health Service requires a certificate issued by the State of origin. These control measures have progressively reduced the incidence of latent infections in California. In 1934, 47, or 23.9 percent, of 196 aviaries were found to harbour latent psittacosis, while in 1941, of 124 establishments only 7 or 5.6 percent, were infected. It is believed that annual retests and a more rigid supervision of dishonest breeders will in time eradicate the infected stocks in California.

Psittacosis in Pigeons and Chickens

The investigation of a fatal case of human psittacosis in California disclosed the important fact that the patient had frequently watched the return of some racing pigeons owned by his son. A blood-serum examination of the 30 pigeons involved was made and 20 gave strong reactions indicative of a present or past infection with the psittacosis virus. The organs of the entire pigeon flock were tested on mice and a virus similar to that of psittacosis was ultimately isolated from one of the pigeons.

While these studies were in progress, the father of another boy who owned a flock of racing pigeons outside Los Angeles contracted psittacosis. In this case, also, a psittacosis virus was demonstrated as being present in the kidneys of an old, emaciated and definitely sick female pigeon in the loft.

In New York, a mother and daughter picked up a sick pigeon; both contracted a disease that was diagnosed as psittacosis at the Rockefeller Hospital. Of 30 pigeons obtained through the courtesy of the New York City Health Department, at least 20 gave positive serum reactions.

A group of pigeons obtained from a dealer in the San Francisco Bay area were held in crowded cages in a damp room. Over a period of a month, 8 birds died. On postmortem examination they showed lesions of emaciation, fibrinous pericarditis (inflammation of the membrane around the heart) and peritonitis (inflammation of the membrane lining the abdominal cavity), spleen tumor and enlarged and engorged livers occasionally studded with small necroses. Since the culture yielded *Salmonella typhimurium* Castellani and Chalmers, the true cause of these deaths was at first not recognized. In view of the observations previously made, an examination of the exudates, or discharges, was instituted and *Microbacterium multiforme psittacosis* was found. The virus was isolated from two of the dead pigeons and serum tests made on the remaining birds indicated that the flock had been heavily exposed to the virus.

The wide distribution in the United States of latent psittacosis in pigeons is further attested by the studies of Pinkerton and Swank,[5] who recovered from the inflamed heart covering of pigeons held on a thiamin-deficient diet a bacterium indistinguishable from *Microbaeterium multiforme psittacosis*. It is amply supported by serum tests which have been recently made on birds from lofts located in various sections of California, South Carolina and Iowa. Between 10 and 50 percent of the tests have produced positive reactions. Although the data are limited, they indicate the widespread existence of a

---

[5] PINKERTON, H., AND SWANK, R.L. RECOVERY OF VIRUS MORPHOLOGICALLY IDENTICAL WITH PSITTACOSIS FROM THIAMIN-DEFICIENT PIGEONS. Soc. Expt. Biol, and Med; 45; 704-706, 1940.

psittacosis infection that possesses a highly adapted parasitism for pigeons. It must be reserved for future studies to determine its spread in the pigeon lofts, its relation to pigeon typhoid, its method of escape from the body, and, in consequence, its potential danger to man. In all probability, it is the direct handling of a sick pigeon that entails a certain risk. Methods of control that may be needed to protect the pigeon-breeding industry will have to be worked out in the future.

Once more in connection with the investigation of a human case of psittacosis, attention was called to the possibility that the high mortality of the chickens on a farm in New Jersey had some definite relationship to the case. Investigations led to the isolation of the psittacosis virus from two chickens from this poultry ranch. The disease agent resembles that found in pigeons in a great many ways. How the infection was brought to the poultry-raising establishment is not known. It is not unlikely that doves or pigeons may have introduced it. As early as 1933, Meyer and Eddie observed the transmission of psittacosis to chickens held in a pen with psittacosis infected parrakeets. The innate susceptibility of the fowl to psittacosis was thus recognized; in the light of the information presented, it must be looked upon as a potentially important poultry disease in the future. From both an economic and a public health point of view, it is imperative that these apparently new infections should receive prompt and detailed investigation.

Chapter 6

MISCELLANEOUS DISEASES OF POULTRY

Hubert Bunyea[1]

[1] *Hubert Bunyea is Veterinarian, Pathological Division, Bureau of Animal Industry.*

This article discusses various diseases and injuries to which poultry are subject, including paratyphoid infection; fowl typhoid; fowl cholera; thrush; aspergillosis; favus; epidemic tremor; avian tuberculosis; poisoning; and bumblefoot, sod disease and other forms of lameness. The author ends with a set of general recommendations for keeping poultry healthy.

Paratyphoid Infection

Fowls are susceptible to numerous infections attributable to some member of the paratyphoid group of organisms, of the genus *Salmonella*. Among the principal avian paratyphoid infections are those caused by *S. anatum* in ducks and by *S. aertrycke* in chickens, ducklings, pigeons and other species (typhimurium). *S. enteritidis* infection of chicks and ducks is prevalent in Europe but not common in the United States.

Paratyphoid infection is characterized by inflammation of the intestines (enteritis), lack of appetite (inappetence), unthriftiness and diarrhea. The mortality rate is variable. This is essentially a disease of young birds. In adult birds it seldom occurs in acute form, but it may occur with low-grade symptoms, either sporadically or as an epizootic (corresponding to an epidemic of a human disease). In pigeons it is characterized by symptoms of inflammation of the lining of the stomach and intestines (gastroenteritis) and by the formation of abscesses around the joints (periarticular abscesses), especially the wing joints (paratyphoid arthritis), which interfere seriously with flying. The abscesses tend to recover without surgical treatment and flying may be resumed.

The frequency with which the *Salmonella* organism is recovered from ovaries indicates that the infection is probably in some instances transmitted through the egg. Infection may also occur in other organs of the body and be disseminated in the droppings.

Paratyphoid infections are difficult to control. The use of blood tests similar to the test successful used for diagnosis and control of pullorum disease has not been found practical. The use of hygienic measures in the hatching and rearing of the young is of paramount importance in controlling the disease. Sometimes, however, it is extremely difficult to apply such measures in pigeon husbandry, for example, the squabs must be fed and reared by the adult pigeons. If it is noted that certain adult birds are particularly unsuccessful in rearing their young on account of paratyphoid infection, such birds should not be used for breeding, or, if they are especially valuable, their eggs might be hatched and the squabs reared by healthy foster parents.

Eggs and poultry affected by paratyphoid infections should not be used as food. In Europe food poisoning has occurred in numerous instances from meringues, mayonnaise, custards and other articles containing uncooked or partially cooked duck eggs. In the United States one or two instances of such poisoning have served to emphasize the advisability of thoroughly cooking duck eggs originating from flocks known to be or suspected of being affected with paratyphoid infections. The flesh of squabs harbouring paratyphoid infection, if incompletely cooked, may also be the cause of food poisoning of human beings.

Fowl Typhoid

Fowl typhoid occurs sporadically in almost every part of the United States. It attacks chickens, turkeys, pigeons and other domestic species. Being a form of bacteriemic infection [2] caused by *Shigella gallinarum*, it somewhat resembles fowl cholera in its symptoms and course. Mortality is not so high as in fowl cholera, however and in general the condition is not of major importance, particularly in chickens. The decline of the disease among chickens probably results, at least in part, from the fact that typhoid carriers are detected by the blood test for pullorum disease and are removed along with the pullorum carriers. Typhoid in turkeys is increasing in importance.

In the absence of a remedy or a dependable vaccine for typhoid, the condition must be controlled largely through the application of sanitary measures. No reliable statistics are available concerning mortality among poultry due to various causes, but this disease is not now an important factor in poultry raising.

Fowl Cholera

Fowl cholera is an infectious disease caused by the organism *Pasteurella avicida*. It affects all domesticated fowl but is most serious in chickens. It is manifested by intestinal disturbances, depression and a high mortality. The disease assumes both the acute and, chronic forms. Chronic cases may become carriers and perpetuate the infection from season to season. Outside the body of the carrier, the infection is easily destroyed by sanitary measures and by the natural elements. In the absence of any dependable means of immunizing susceptible birds or curing sick ones, sanitation has been the principal defence against fowl cholera for many years. A whole blood agglutination test has recently been developed which detects fowl cholera carriers, thus making it possible to remove the source of perpetuation of the infection. It is thought that the application of this test during a chronic outbreak or at the subsidence of an acute outbreak will permit the detection of the carrier birds and that their removal will break the cycle of the infection in the flock. The test has not yet gained wide acceptance, however and has had only limited trials.

Fowl cholera is not limited in its occurrence to any particular geographical location. It is probably most prevalent in the Middle West and it is a serious problem at poultry-fattening plants and

---

[2] A bacteriemic infection is one characterized by the presence of living bacteria in the blood stream.

among feeder poultry in transit by railroad to eastern markets but not in the industry generally. No figures are available as to the losses caused by this disease.

Mycosis

Mycosis is a disease caused by fungus growths. Fungi attack the skin, respiratory tract and digestive tract of chickens. The most serious type of mycosis is that which affects the digestive tract. Known as thrush or moniliasis and caused by the fungus *Saccharomyces albicans*, it affects chickens, pigeons, turkeys and geese. Gray or white patches form on the mucous membranes of the gastric tract and sometimes enlarge and run together. A discharge runs from the mouth. Loss of appetite, weakness and emaciation ensue and there is a progressive diarrhoea, with green droppings. Mortality runs high in the affected birds and production is curtailed in those that survive.

Medicinal treatment in the form of mild antiseptics may be applied to visible lesions, but the disease, if deep-seated, is beyond the reach of drugs. Clean houses, clean drinking fountains, feed that is free from molds and dry litter all aid in the prevention or control of the disease. It is not of major economic importance and probably does not occur to any great extent in well-managed establishments.

Preparatory to medicinal treatment, the accessible thrush deposits in the mouth and larynx of the affected bird should be removed with forceps, after which the ulcers should be painted with a mixture of 4 parts of glycerin and 1 part of tincture of iodine. Thrush of the crop may be treated by washing out the crop with a 2 percent solution of boric acid, using a fountain syringe.

Mycosis of the Air Passages (Aspergillosis)

Mycosis of the air passages may occur in any species of fowl but is particularly prevalent among waterfowl and zoo birds. It is caused by the green mold *Aspergillus fumigatus* and sometimes by the black mold *A. niger*.

The disease assumes the form of chronic progressive dyspnea (laboured breathing) attended with unthriftiness and emaciation, Mucous rales–a gurgling sound in the breathing–occur when the bird exhales. These and the usual mouth-breathing (gasping) symptoms may be mistaken for evidences of avian diphtheria, laryngo- tracheitis, bronchitis, or coryza. Aspergillosis, however, may be differentiated at autopsy by the appearance of white or dirty-yellowish nodules (small lumps) in the trachea, lungs, or air sacs. In advanced cases these lesions may coalesce into elevated dirty deposits consisting of mold growths in the air passages. Aspergillosis in brooder chicks (brooder pneumonia) may be confused with pullorum disease, which sometimes affects the lungs of baby chicks, producing dyspneic and pneumonic manifestations. Aspergillosis of young chicks is rapidly and invariably fatal. In older birds the condition assumes the more chronic form, but there are no recoveries. Medicinal treatment or vaccination is of no known value in combating the condition. The only procedure that can be recommended as having any prospect of controlling aspergillosis is the practice of strict sanitation. Moldy feeds and moldy litter must be removed; floors, nests, dropping boards and feed and water containers should be cleaned and disinfected; and clean litter and unspoiled feed should be provided.

Feed bags that have become damp and moldy are a possible source of the disease and should be destroyed. Feed should be purchased in new bags and stored in such a way that molds and dampness cannot occur. The feeding of wet mashes necessitates scrupulous care in the daily cleansing of the feed receptacles. Left-over wet mash should be discarded beyond the reach of the flock. The sick birds should be segregated or, better still, destroyed so they cannot spread the infection. Those that die should be burned or otherwise disposed of properly.

Mycosis of the Skin (Favus, White Comb, Avian Mycotic Dermatitis)

Favus is caused by the fungus *Lophophyton gallinae,* which is readily transmitted from bird to bird and is also said to be infectious to human beings. It is manifested by the formation of grayish-white growths or crusts on the unfeathered head parts of the affected bird. If it spreads to the feathered part, the feathers break off and the disease becomes increasingly difficult to control. Birds so affected had better be destroyed. When only the unfeathered parts of the body are affected, the daily application of tincture of iodine to the, lesions has been recommended. Greater success has been reported, however, from applying formalized petrolatum, which is prepared by adding 5 percent (by weight) of commercial formalin to melted petrolatum and shaking these together in a tightly closed container until the petrolatum has congealed. One application of formalized petrolatum is said to have effected a cure in nearly all cases treated. *Rubber gloves should be worn during its preparation and administration.*

Infectious Avian Encephalomyelitis

Infectious avian encephalomyelitis (epidemic tremor) occurs in chicks 1 to 2 days up to 2 to 3 weeks old. Fifty percent or more of the chicks in a flock may be affected. Many are likely to recover, but others may continue to manifest some tremor symptoms for a time.

The practice usually recommended is to finish surviving chicks quickly for early marketing as broilers or fryers. Under favourable living conditions, the recovered and slowly convalescing birds may mature and may become normally productive of eggs and healthy chicks. They may, however, turn out to be carriers of the infection, which they may transmit to their offspring.

The disease does not usually affect every hatch but may disappear during the hatching season only to return unexpectedly, recurring sporadically from time to time with varying degrees of severity.

The disease is disseminated through contact among the brood. It may also be spread through contact in the incubator and there is some scientific evidence to indicate that infection may be handed down from parent to offspring through the egg. In this way epidemic tremor may be broadcast to remote areas through the dispersal of an infected or exposed hatch of chicks. Fortunately some strains of chickens appear to possess more resistance to the disease than others.

Avian Tuberculosis

Tuberculosis is a chronic infectious disease which affects practically all species of domesticated birds and many species of wild birds in captivity. It is manifested by the formation of nodules in various organs, such as the liver, spleen, kidneys and heart muscle and along the mesentery and intestinal tract. The seriousness of the tuberculosis problem in connection with poultry, the distribution of the disease, the use of the tuberculin test and the preventive measures are discussed in the article on Tuberculosis, page 246. It is necessary here to add only a few points to that discussion.

The clinical diagnosis of avian tuberculosis is difficult because maney of the symptoms, such as emaciation, dejection, articular lameness of legs or wings, paleness and diarrhoea, are common to other conditions. However, the occurrence of numerous cases showing one or more of such symptoms, along with a history of occasional mortality in the flock, strongly suggests tuberculosis infection. An early symptom is emaciation of the breast muscles and this progresses to the point where no flesh separates the skin and bone. The bird continues to eat well and the temperature remains normal until the approach of death, when it becomes subnormal. Autopsies of such birds show an almost complete absence of body or visceral fat.

The lameness occurring in an advanced stage of the disease is occasioned by purulent swellings of the affected articulations, or joints. These swellings may rupture and exude a cheesy pus. The head parts are strikingly pale, withered and dry. Listlessness and weakness are progressive. A greenish or yellowish diarrhoea develops and aggravates the weakened condition of the birds. The feathers if assume a ruffled, unkempt appearance as a result of the bird's weakness and neglect in preening itself.

Tuberculous lesions found in the carcass include large or small tumorlike masses within the liver, spleen, kidney, ovaries, peritoneum, intestinal tract, joints and elsewhere. The occurrence of such lesions is not, however, conclusive as a diagnosis of tuberculosis. The final proof is the microscopic demonstration of the presence of the organism of the disease.

The tuberculin test is, in general, reliable and it is useful within certain limits. The cost of the test and the labour of applying it, although moderate, must be taken into consideration, especially when planning to test flocks of no more than average value. Whether or not the tuberculin test is applied, it is important to obtain a diagnosis when the disease is suspected.

Since avian tuberculosis is not amenable to medicinal treatment, the only method of control is the slaughter of all reactors to tuberculin or all clinically suspicious cases of the disease. Where the infection appears to have taken a firm hold, it is frequently desirable to destroy the entire flock; although, if the birds are of exceptional breeding value, it may be advisable in rare cases to preserve them long enough to obtain a few hatching eggs to perpetuate the strain. Such eggs must be hatched and the resulting chicks reared under the most hygienic conditions.

After an outbreak of tuberculosis, strict sanitary measures, including disinfection, should be taken, as discussed at pages 126-127. Only after the premises have been completely freed of the infection will it be safe to introduce new stock from healthy sources.

The practice of disposing of all birds when they are about 16 or 18 months of age tends to reduce to a minimum the chances of having dangerous cases of tuberculosis on the place, since it is known that as a rule the disease develops very slowly in the growing bird.

Common Forms of Poisoning of Poultry

Limber-Neck (Botulism)

The toxic disease known as limber-neck, or botulism, of chickens is characterized primarily by the dysphagia (difficult swallowing) caused by paralysis of the pharynx, lack of appetite and a paralysis of the neck muscles which makes it impossible for the bird to raise or control its head.

Botulism is caused by eating feed or other material which has been contaminated with the organism *Clostridium botulinum* and on which this germ has multiplied and elabourated its toxic byproducts. Decomposed flesh and the maggots of flies which have bred on it are considered probable sources of botulinus poisoning. Ducks frequenting the western marshlands have died in great numbers from botulism.

Early symptoms of botulism include lassitude, drowsiness and leg weakness. The fowl first loses the ability to stand on its feet and then the power to hold up its head. It finally assumes a posture of extreme prostration from which it cannot be aroused. The feathers become loose and are easily shed if the bird is handled. The severity of the symptoms depends on the amount of the toxin swallowed. The paralysis may affect the eyes to the extent of preventing the contraction of the pupils and may also cause a relaxation of the bowels, resulting in diarrhoea.

The course of the disease is fairly rapid, death usually occurring a few hours after the appearance of symptoms.

By the time symptoms are noted, it is usually too late for effective treatment. Birds exposed to the toxin but not yet affected may be given a drench of Epsom salts solution, 1 pound of Epsom salts being used for each 100 birds treated, or about 1 teaspoonful of the crystals, dissolved in water, for each bird. The solution may be introduced into the crop by means of a funnel or fountain syringe to insure complete dosage and prompt action. Botulinus antitoxin, types A and C, may be given intraperitoneally–injected into the lining of the abdomen. (Type B botulinus toxin does not affect poultry.) The cost of the treatment is prohibitive, however, except for birds of unusual value.

The crops of affected or exposed birds may be emptied and flushed out with fluids or evacuated by surgical incision if the value of the birds justifies such procedure.

When an outbreak of limber-neck occurs, an effort should be made to locate the cause. Decomposed flesh, dead animals and fowls, etc., which may be accessible to poultry, should be burned or buried. Spoiled canned goods used as feed are a prolific source of limber-neck among poultry.

Chemical Poisoning

Poultry are susceptible to chemical poisoning, but they exhibit a tolerance for relatively large doses of some poisonous substances. It is not wise, however, to leave rat poisons containing arsenic, phosphorus, barium carbonate, or other poisonous substances within reach of poultry, or to allow poultry access to orchards, cabbage patches; or other farm areas that have recently been sprayed or dusted with arsenical preparations.

Arsenic is sometimes employed for poisoning locusts or grass-hoppers. Poultry eating a number of such poisoned insects or a quantity of the bait may be poisoned by the arsenic. Chickens sometimes gain access to poison bait containing strychnin intended for poisoning crows or hawks, with disastrous results.

Kamala and nicotine sulfate, sometimes used for ridding poultry of parasites, are dangerous unless used in accordance with directions. Kamala may cause a serious bowel disturbance, with a resultant loss of egg production as well as a decrease in egg weight. Small doses of a well-diluted solution of nicotine sulfate have proved fatal to young chickens.

Other toxic material frequently left within reach of poultry includes fish brine, ice-cream salt, calcium carbide slack from acetylene gas tanks and similar substances. Spent fireworks are dangerous around poultry premises. Instances are on record of children detonating "devil-chasers" in the driveway of the farm home and leaving them there, with the result that early the next morning pullets picked up the sharp gravel from the fireworks in the driveway and within a short time died of phosphorus poisoning.

Satisfactory treatments of poultry for the various kinds of chemical poisoning mentioned are not known.

Rose Chafer Poisoning

Rose chafers are found in great numbers on grapevines, rose bushes and other shrubbery during the spring. Young chickens eat these beetles readily and are fatally poisoned by a relatively small number of them. Some birds may recover from a slight attack of the poisoning. Drowsiness and weakness are the first symptoms, followed by prostration and convulsions. The head is thrown back and the bird utters shrill cries.

No treatment is effective after the poison has begun to act. Birds that have been exposed to the danger may be given Epsom salts or castor oil to hasten the elimination of any beetles swallowed. Young chicks should be restrained from visiting areas infested with rose chafers.

Lameness in Poultry

Poultry may acquire leg lameness and sometimes wing lameness from a variety of causes, environmental, nutritional, infectious and parasitic.

Lameness Due to Environmental Conditions

Injuries

Young chicks sometimes get their feet or hock joints caught in the meshes of wire-cloth battery-brooder floors. As a precaution against such accidents it is well to use wire cloth of sufficiently close mesh so that the legs or feet of chicks are not likely to become ensnared.

Fowls of any age living where the winters are cold may freeze their toes and feet. If sufficiently frost-bitten, the toes will become swollen and sore, then gangrenous and finally drop off leaving the foot tender and crippled. There is no cure for seriously frosted feet. The obvious preventive measure is to confine the fowls to comfortable living quarters with warm, dry floors and plenty of litter.

Bumblefoot

Bumblefoot is a swelling of the feet of poultry caused by an accumulation of a cheesy exudate, or discharge. Various explanations have been offered for its occurrence. It has long been believed that injury caused by jumping from high roosts to hard floors was responsible for this condition, but its occurrence where roosts are low and floors are well bedded with litter throws doubt upon that theory. It is probable that, through briar wounds and otherwise, infection gains entry into the tissues of the foot and sets up the production of pus in the underlying tissues, causing the bird great pain as well as lameness.

Staphylococcus aureus, the yellow-pus organism, has frequently been isolated from bumblefoot lesions and is considered the probable cause in some cases. An acid-fast organism resembling *Mycobacterium tuberculosis avium* has been demonstrated microscopically to be present in this condition, but its significance as a causative factor has not been established.

The treatment of bumblefoot should include all possible provisions for relieving the suffering of the affected birds. Low roosts and well-bedded floors are helpful. The abscesses may be evacuated by removing the scabs from the pad of the foot and the between the toes spaces and extracting the cheesy pus by pressure and the use of forceps. In advanced cases it may be necessary to lance the foot to remove the pus completely. The cavity may then be irrigated with some mild but effective antiseptic, such as 5 percent phenol or full-strength hydrogen peroxide solution, after which the cavity may be packed with pads of cotton soaked in a similar solution and bandaged with gauze and adhesive tape to keep the wound clean. The treatment should be repeated at 2 to 3 day intervals until evidence of healing appears.

A type of bumblefoot caused by a deficiency of vitamin A has been described.

Sod Disease

Sod disease is a vesicular dermatitis (an inflammation of the skin characterized by small swellings filled with fluid) of young chicks and occasionally older fowls ranging in early summer on unbroken prairie land. Blisters and swelling of the feet, culminating in scabs, eventually cause lameness. Parts of or even whole toes may slough off. Recovered birds may develop misshapen toes. The eyelids may stick together and the birds may be unable to find their feed.

The disease is economically important not only because of rather high mortality in young birds but also because of the permanent disability caused by chronic foot trouble in recovered cases.

No cause or cure for the disease is known, but it can be easily prevented by excluding the birds from unplowed prairie land.

Lameness Due to Faulty Nutrition

Nutritional diseases of poultry are discussed in detail in another part of this report. The types of lameness that may be classified as of nutritional origin include articular gout, polyneuritis, rickets, slipped tendon (perosis), nutritional encephalomalacia and nutritional paralysis and curled-toe disease.

One of the forms of gout consists of swollen and painful joints of the legs or wings caused by the depositing of urates in the articular regions, rendering movement difficult and increasing the danger of starvation. Although the cause of gout is not clear in all cases, it is believed at times to be due to a prolonged feeding of high protein rations. Lack of exercise and factors affecting the proper function of the kidneys are also possibly involved in the origin and development of gout.

The swollen joints, if opened at autopsy, are found to contain a yellowish exudate consisting of waste matter from the kidneys. Similar chalky deposits may be found in the kidneys, which are usually pale and swollen. The surface of the heart, liver, spleen and mesentery may also present a pearly chalklike appearance due to urate deposits (salts of uric acid) and may reveal a marked absence of visceral fat.

From the dietetic standpoint, the occurrence of gout in a flock suggests the advisability of a reduction of protein to a level of not more than 10 percent of the total ration and an increase in the proportion of bulky green feeds. The entire flock may be put on a saline purge consisting in the administration of a solution containing one-third of a teaspoonful of Epsom salts crystals per hen. The painful swellings in the vicinity of articulations may be lanced and the urates evacuated, after which the incision may be dressed with a healing ointment such as zinc oxide ointment and bandaged to keep out contamination.

Lameness Due to Infections

The principal form of lameness due to infection is fowl paralysis.

Paratyphoid arthritis occurring specifically in pigeons infected with *Salmonella typhimurium* is discussed in connection with paratyphoid infections.

Lameness from Fowl Cholera

Like avian tuberculosis, fowl cholera tends to form localized foci of infection. Common locations are in the articular regions of the legs or wings.

Outbreaks of the chronic form of fowl cholera may be characterized by a number of cases of lameness in the flock. An examination of the lame birds may disclose a soft or doughy lump on the joint of the affected member. The abscess will be found to be filled with pus as a result of localization of the cholera infection at that point. The presence of the active infection in these lesions may be demonstrated by labouratory procedures.

No treatment for lameness from fowl cholera infection can be recommended. Birds so affected are a menace and should be destroyed.

Staphylococcic Arthritis

In addition to being a cause of bumblefoot, the pus-producing organism *Staphylococcus aureus*, through infection of the joints, causes a number of other conditions resulting in lameness of the feet, legs, or wings of various species of birds.

Staphylococcic arthritis occurs in chickens, ducks, geese, turkeys, pigeons, pheasants and possibly other species. The common symptoms in all species are lameness and swelling of the affected joints. Autopsy findings may vary from local abscesses to the erosion of articular surfaces of the bones and pus in the tendon sheaths and bones. Mortality is relatively high.

Treatment is palliative, giving relief only and consists in providing comfortable housing conditions, with feed and water easily accessible to the sick birds. Separation of the affected individuals contributes to their comfort and may help to check the spread of the disease. Sanitation about the premises, including cleanliness of feed and water supply, should not be overlooked. No medicinal treatment can be recommended.

Lameness from Parasitic Infestation

Chickens, turkeys, pheasants, partridges and caged birds are susceptible to infestation by a parasitic itch mite (*Cnemidocoptes mutans*), which causes the condition known as scaly leg, discussed in the article on Poultry Mites.

Keeping Poultry Healthy

Proper location of the poultry house will do much toward keeping a flock healthy. The poultry quarters should be on light, preferably sandy, well-drained soil and should be provided with some trees or shelters for shade. The house should face opposite the direction from which storms ordinarily come.

Clean, comfortable, well-ventilated and spacious poultry houses, abundant and nourishing feeds and clean water in clean receptacles help keep fowls in good physical condition; when these things are provided, no medicine is needed to keep poultry well and productive. Without such provisions, no medicinal treatment will insure the maintenance of health.

In brooder houses, young fowls require some warmth under the hovers, but only enough not to become chilled. Too much heat is probably as unfavourable as too little. Ventilation is essential, when coal or oil heat is used, since chicks in poorly ventilated brooder houses may be killed by an accumulation of carbon monoxide gas. The floor space should not be crowded and as the chicks grow they should from time to time be given additional room. By degrees, depending on the advance of milder weather and the State of development of the birds, artificial heat should be gradually diminished.

Feed hoppers and water fountains of a size and shape to provide space for fowls of any age should be supplied; otherwise, some birds will monopolize the privileges and others, perhaps small and unthrifty to start with, will be crowded out.

Growing stock may be reared to maturity on open range provided sufficient area is available so that the houses or range shelters may be moved at frequent intervals. Sufficient ground around the shelter may be enclosed so that the birds may range for a week or more. Grass sod makes an excellent range for young poultry, but the location should be changed before the sod is bare or the ground polluted. As the birds grow additional space becomes necessary and this can be provided by taking out the males at about 8 weeks of age.

When the breeders are taken off the range, weaklings and unthrifty birds should be rigidly culled out. The laying houses, including floors, dropping boards and nests, should be in good condition and thoroughly cleaned and disinfected, aired out and thoroughly dried and the floors should be covered with clean litter for the new occupants. Provision should be made for correct ventilation. Feed and water receptacles should be clean and in good working condition. Large laying flocks had best be divided into smaller breeding units, not only from the standpoint of matings and as good husbandry practice, but also as an aid to proper hygiene. Pullets off the range should be housed separately from old hens. Under no circumstances should birds of different species be housed together.

The windows of laying houses should be covered with mesh wire to keep out free-flying birds. Fly screening is even better, since flies and mosquitoes are carriers of poultry-disease infections. The doors also should be screened. Poultry hucksters, feed and remedy salesmen and other transients should be positively excluded from poultry houses and their vicinity. In disease-ridden localities it is good policy to refrain from showing neighbours or visitors around poultry premises or, if this cannot be tactfully avoided, to provide them with clean overshoes. Where poultry diseases exist in one part of the establishment or in neighbouring flocks, it is suggested that at the door of the poultry houses cocomats be set in shallow concrete depressions and be kept soaked with a diluted cresol compound solution, carbolic acid, or stock dip. Persons entering the houses may thus easily wipe and disinfect the soles of their footwear at one operation. The lye solutions recommended elsewhere in this article for disinfecting purposes might be injurious to shoes.

New birds purchased for breeding or show purposes, as well as birds returning from poultry exhibitions or egg-laying contests, should be kept under quarantine for observation for a period of 2 to 4 weeks before being placed with the flock. Should there be evidence of disease during this period, competent advice should be sought concerning the disposal of such birds or others exposed to them.

The occurrence of infectious disease in a flock calls for prompt and decisive action. The sick birds should be carefully separate from the healthy ones and if possible the healthy birds should be moved to clean comfortable quarters. If this is not practicable, the sick ones must be taken out and the place promptly cleaned and disinfected as thoroughly as possible, the healthy birds during this time being temporarily moved out to a place where no diseased poultry have been. After each room is cleaned and disinfected, new dry litter should be placed on the floor and then the flock may be readmitted. The healthy birds should be closely observed for the possible appearance of new cases of disease.

The advisability of keeping the sick birds in separate quarters for medicinal treatment is very doubtful. It is usually better to destroy them since sick chickens seldom respond to treatment and may only be a means of perpetuating infection on the premises. The carcasses of fowls that die from disease should be autopsied, if at all, by a competent diagnostician. In any event such carcasses should be, completely burned or buried deep in the ground.

Preparatory to disinfecting poultry houses, all nesting, litter, manure and other contaminated material and movable equipment should be removed. Dust and cobwebs should be swept from the ceilings window sills and ledges. Beginning with the ceiling and taking in all surfaces, the entire room from top to bottom should be thoroughly sprayed with a suitable germicidal solution. Numerous disinfecting substances are satisfactory for this operation.[3] For general purposes a satisfactory solution may be prepared by

---

[3] The reader is referred to Farmers' Bulletin 926, Some Common Disinfectants, and Farmers' Bulletin 954, The Disinfection of Stables, as well as to Disinfection and Disinfectants, in this Yearbook, p. 179.

dissolving 1 pound of commercial lye containing 94 percent of sodium hydroxide and 2½ pounds of water-slaked lime in 5½ gallons of water. It should be strained through a fine wire screen to remove particles of lime which might otherwise clog the sprayer. Any type of sprayer may be used to apply the disinfectant, but one that generates enough air pressure to drive the solution with considerable force onto the surface to be disinfected is especially effective. All surfaces should be thoroughly wet with the solution, which should also be forced into all cracks and corners. The white residue on the surface that has received the treatment will indicate spots that have been missed. The unused solution should be tightly covered to prevent deterioration. The ground around the poultry house may be disinfected with the same solution, using ½ to 1 gallon for each square yard to be disinfected. The yard must, however, be thoroughly cleaned of trash and refuse beforehand.

Because of the caustic nature of lye solutions, the following precautions should be observed: *The operator should protect his person and clothing by wearing rubber boots, coat, hat and gloves. He should also protect his eyes with goggles.* Lye solutions should not be used on painted surfaces or fabric curtains. The spray apparatus should be thoroughly flushed out with clean water after use to avoid damage to leather or fabric gaskets, fabric-lined hose, etc.

A single exception is made to the recommendation of lye solution as a disinfectant. It has been found that it does not destroy the germs of tuberculosis. To combat that infection, the usual preparatory measures are taken, after which the premises and utensils are thoroughly sprayed with a material such as compound solution of creosol or a permitted saponified creosol solution in 3 percent dilution, or carbolic acid in 5 percent dilution. Some other germicides also are known to be effective against *Mycobacterium tuberculosis avium*.

A final suggestion concerning the prevention of diseases in poultry: It is a good idea to provide for a competent periodic inspection service on the health of the flock, including expert advice on the hygiene of the surroundings. Such service cannot be satisfactorily given by itinerant "poultry specialists," who probably have no reliable recommendation and all too frequently have something to sell. The local veterinarian, on the other hand, has qualified himself for the task of controlling poultry diseases and may be looked to with, confidence to make clinical examinations, apply diagnostic tests, administer vaccines and remedies and suggest sanitary measures calculated to cope with whatever disease problem may confront the poultryman. The staffs of many State agricultural experiment stations are also in a position to render similar services. Poultrymen would save themselves considerable financial and other losses if they would obtain competent diagnosis and advice on disease problems instead of giving undue heed to the advice of unqualified strangers or even to that of well-meaning but uninformed neighbours.

Chapter 7

INTERNAL PARASITES OF POULTRY

Everett E. Wehr & John F. Christensen[1]

[1] *Everett E. Wehr is Zoologist and John F. Christensen is Associate Protozoologist, Zoological Division, Bureau of Animal Industry.*

A thorough account of the principal parasites of poultry in the United States, including practical measures for preventing some of the heavy annual losses from this source.

James E. Rice, formerly head of the Poultry Husbandry Department of Cornell University, who has been called the father of poultry husbandry in the United States, once made the statement that there was no way to save the poultry industry except through a scientific approach to the control of poultry diseases. The significance of this statement becomes apparent with the realisation that losses from poultry diseases in the United States have been estimated by Government authorities to be approximately 100 million dollars annually.

That the presence of disease has been responsible for the curtailment of poultry raising in many areas cannot be questioned. A few years ago poultrymen in many sections of the United States were forced to abandon the raising of turkeys because of the prevalence of blackhead, caused by a protozoan parasite. Only a drastic change in poultry-husbandry practices made turkey production again a profitable enterprise in these areas.

Farmers are losing 18.8 percent of their poultry because of disease, or 1 out of every 5 birds, according to C.M. Ferguson of the University of Ohio. This is a tremendous loss, since statistics indicate that chickens are kept on 85 percent of the farms in the United States at the present time.

Internal parasitism is usually more insidious and therefore not so noticeable as specific diseases, many of which are deadly in their effects and spectacular in nature, put parasites constitute a real menace to successful poultry raising. Unlike bacterial diseases, the majority of the parasitic diseases do not result in early fatalities. The protozoan diseases, blackhead and coccidiosis, are exceptions, since the destruction of the intestinal mucous membrane in the former and of the liver tissue in the latter are attended by a high rate of mortality.

Poultry raisers are demanding more and better control measures for both parasites and diseases. Though only a few satisfactory drugs for the removal of poultry parasites have been found, practical and reliable control measures are not lacking. Sanitation, when properly carried out, has proved to be one of the most effective and practical means of reducing parasitism in poultry flocks.

Since measures for the control of internal parasites in poultry are largely preventive and apply to almost the whole group of parasites, they will be discussed first in this article. The little that can be done in the way of curative treatment will also be included in the first part of the article. Descriptions of the large numbers of poultry parasites and the injuries they cause will follow the section on control.

Control of Poultry Parasites

Many species of parasites must spend a part of their developmental cycle outside the body of the host or they cannot continue to exist. In the case of poultry parasites, with few exceptions, the stage away from the bird is spent in the feces. Some of the protozoan parasites, however, spend this developmental stage in the blood stream and these parasites are therefore not eliminated through any of the body openings of the host. Their escape from the body depends on their being removed by bloodsucking insects.

In their infective stages, parasites are introduced into susceptible hosts in a number of ways:

(1) By means of contaminated litter and soil.
(2) By means of contaminated food and water.
(3) By means of carriers; birds that have had a light infection or have survived a more severe one may carry the organisms within their intestinal tracts for long periods of time and spread the parasites in their discharges.
(4) By intermediate hosts; insects such as flies, mosquitoes and beetles, or other low forms of animal life such as snails and slugs, in which a part of the development of the parasite takes place, are eaten by susceptible hosts and as a result infection is set up.
(5) By mechanical means; animals and human beings may carry infective material on their feet and thus spread the parasites from one pen to another–attendants have been known to carry infective material from an infected pen to a sanitary one; contaminated chicken coops and other equipment may be a source of infection when carelessly moved from place to place or used for healthy birds.

Prevention Versus Cure

The old adage that an ounce of prevention is worth a pound of cure is just as applicable to poultry parasites as it is to human diseases. After a disease has once gained a foothold in a flock, far more time and money are usually spent in getting rid of the disease than would have been necessary to keep the premises free of it. In addition, the mortality may be high before the disease is finally checked.

Preventive measures include sanitation, disinfection, hygiene and management.

Sanitation and Hygiene

Sanitation means establishing an environment in which the possibility of infection with disease-producing organisms is reduced to a minimum.

The first essential is the proper selection of the poultry site. The soil should be of a sandy or gravelly nature in order to provide for good drainage. To take advantage of natural drainage, the site should preferably be located on a gentle slope. If the lay of the land or the nature of the soil renders natural drainage impossible, artificial drainage must be resorted to. Since moisture is essential to the development of most parasites in their free-living stages, the presence of surface water, which the birds are apt to drink, must be regarded as unhealthful. Pools of water in the poultry yards should be immediately filled in or drained.

Poultry houses or shelters are essential for the protection of the birds against inclement weather, including rain, storms and extremes of temperature. The excreta, or body wastes, of the birds which collect in the houses or shelters must be properly handled, or they may serve as a source of infection with parasites and other diseases. Irrespective of the type of poultry house built, it is of the utmost importance that it possess certain features of design and arrangement to facilitate cleaning and to keep the birds well and strong. The floors and walls should be constructed of material that is impervious to moisture and easy to clean and will exclude vermin of all types. Floors of dirt or wood are seriously objectionable because they are difficult to clean and disinfect; concrete floors are much more desirable. The roosts and nests should be simply constructed so that they may be taken apart easily for cleaning and disinfecting. (See Farmers' Bulletin 1070 (*10*)[2]. The house should be so constructed as to insure the entrance of an abundance of direct sunlight, which is important to the health of the fowls as well as destructive to bacteria and certain parasites.

The hygienic condition of poultry yards is of tremendous importance to the health of the birds. It is not so convenient to collect and dispose of body wastes in the poultry runs as in the houses. For this reason, the small overcrowded poultry runs too frequently observed are apt to receive a larger amount of wastes than the ground can adequately take care of. When a disease is once introduced in such a place, it quickly becomes epizootic, that is, like an epidemic among human beings and soon all the birds have contracted it. This condition exists on many farms in the United States and because of the prevalence of disease under such conditions, the individual farm flock rarely pays for itself.

Permanent Quarters or Rotation

Keeping birds on the same ground year after year will ultimately

---

[2] Italic numbers in parentheses refer to Literature Cited.

cause the soil to become a more or less continual hotbed of infection if parasitized or diseased birds are present in the flock. The eggs of parasites are known to live in the soil from year to year and contaminated soil serves as an important source of infection for the intermediate hosts of poultry parasites.

What is the remedy for such a situation? The course that a poultryman may choose depends very largely on the size of the flock, the available space for rearing the birds, the amount of money that can be allotted for poultry equipment and the type of soil. If only a small area of land is available, it may be best to raise the birds in confinement. This system has the advantage that the birds may occupy the same quarters year after year. In order to provide adequate sunlight, a small wire-covered sun porch may be constructed in front of the house, or there may be a small fenced-in yard covered with cinders or other porous material.

Where a considerable area of land is available for poultry raising, the practice of rotating the fowls has been followed with reasonably good success. This system consists of using enclosed poultry yards which are occupied by the birds intermittently in order to prevent excessive contamination. The four-yard system is the one most widely advocated and is probably the one best suited for general farm practice. A plot of land–the acreage depends on the number of birds to be raised, figuring about 650 to 800 birds per acre–is fenced and cross fenced so as to have four equal-sized pens. The shelter or house is located in the center of the plot and built with a door opening directly into each pen. The birds are placed in lot No. 1, kept therefore a month or two and then moved into lot No. 2. The practice of moving the birds at regular intervals from one pen to another is continued until all four pens have been occupied, when the birds are again placed in pen No. 1. Immediately following the removal of the birds from one of the pens, the ground should be prepared and planted to some green crop or left idle to undergo self-sterilization. In the latter case the contaminated soil is left undisturbed so that the sun, wind and cold can act directly on the parasites present in it. Some poultrymen plant the lots to a permanent crop, such as alfalfa. Such a crop furnishes abundant green feed for the growing birds and this makes it less likely that they will pick up contaminated material from the soil. The house and adjacent grounds should be cleaned at least once a week and oftener if necessary.

Manure Disposal

Every poultry owner is faced with the problem of disposing of the body wastes from his birds in a sanitary manner. To allow the excreta to accumulate in large quantities either in the house or in the yard is to bring into operation the law of nature that no species of animal can exist for very long in intimate contact with its own body wastes without endangering its health through the contraction of disease. Wild birds and animals are not restricted in their range as are the species raised in more or less confinement, hence wild creatures are less apt to pick up infections from their excretions.

Under present conditions in the poultry industry it is often necessary to raise several thousand birds together and proper steps must be taken to remove the body wastes at frequent intervals and to dispose of them in a sanitary manner if mortality from disease is to be kept at a low level. The body wastes from farm flocks can readily be disposed of by having them hauled to the fields and spread thinly over the land for use as fertilizer. Poultry manure, when properly handled, is an excellent fertilizer for garden and field crops. The body wastes from flocks raised in back yards or in communities where poultry raising is intensively practiced cannot be so easily disposed of as on the farm and must be taken care of in some other way. In some heavily populated areas, poultry raisers have been known to store the manure from their flocks in one or more centrally located storage sheds and sell it. Poultry manure usually retails for a very good price.

To properly preserve the fertilizing value of poultry manure it must be stored in a suitable screened in shed with a cement floor and a roof to keep out rain and snow. Manure stored in this manner is also protected from flying and crawling insects and other forms of animal life that may serve as carriers or intermediate hosts of poultry parasites. Just that effect the storage of poultry manure in piles has on the livability of the eggs of poultry parasites and of coccidial oöcysts has not been definitely determined.

Different Types of Poultry Should be Raised Seprately

It has been demonstrated, repeatedly that in order to prevent the spread of parasitic and other poultry diseases the different types of poultry should be raised separately and in small flocks.

Observations have shown that turkeys serve as carriers of gapeworms and transmit gapeworm disease to little chicks, while older chickens are almost entirely resistant to gapeworm infection under range conditions. On the other hand, Tyzzer (*46*) shows that chickens carry the organisms of blackhead in their intestinal tracts and young turkeys may contract the disease by exposure to infected chickens or to areas infected by them and usually die in large numbers from the disease. Only in exceptional cases do the chickens show symptoms of the disease and infected chickens usually recover and remain carriers of the organisms for an indefinite period.

It is also dangerous for chickens to associate with pigeons. Levine (*34*) was successful in producing severe experimental infections in chickens with the pigeon capillarid, *Capillaria columbae*. Wehr (*52a*) has reported that chickens heavily infected with *C. columbae* showed symptoms of emaciation, diarrhea and listlessness and that such an infection usually resulted in death.

What to Do in Case of An Outbreak

In case of an outbreak of a poultry disease, an early diagnosis is essential in order that the proper control measures may be employed. Unfortunately, in many places the services of a poultry-disease diagnostician or a competent veterinarian are not available. In such cases, the State agricultural experiment station should be consulted immediately as to the advisability of shipping birds to its poultry department or veterinary science department for a diagnosis. Should it be necessary to ship sick birds to a distant diagnostic labouratory, it may be several days before a reply is received. In the meantime, losses may continue and the disease, if acute in character, may gain such a foothold that control measures, when finally applied, will be of little use. Since it is urgent that the disease be checked as soon as possible after its appearance, it is suggested that the following first-aid measures be put into effect immediately in an attempt to control it before it reaches epizootic proportions.

The first requirement in bringing an outbreak of disease under control is to remove all visibly sick birds from the flock, confine them in a room or house separate from the healthy birds and burn the carcasses of any birds that have died. The healthy birds should if possible be moved to a clean house and clean grounds, but if this is impossible, the body wastes that have accumulated in the house should be disposed of in a sanitary manner and the house and all its equipment should be thoroughly cleaned and disinfected with some suitable disinfectant, such as hot water or hot lye solution. As soon as the house and equipment have been cleaned and disinfected, the healthy birds should be put back in the house and confined there until the symptoms have subsided in the sick birds. During this period of confinement, the healthy birds should be watched carefully and any of them that become sick should be removed immediately and placed with the sick birds. The houses occupied by both the healthy and sick birds should be thoroughly cleaned daily, preferably dry-cleaned and the litter burned. In case of diarrhea, a mild laxative should be given to all the birds. For flock treatment, 1 pound of Epsom salts dissolved in about 2 gallons of water will make enough medicated liquid for 100 birds. The birds should be kept warm and be disturbed as little as possible and crowding should be avoided. The feed should be placed in sanitary hoppers and the watering devices protected with wire frames, so that the birds will have less chance to contaminate the drinking water. If the same person must tend both the sick and the healthy birds, the sick birds should be attended to last in order to prevent the mechanical transfer of the causative agent of the disease to the healthy birds. The attendant should be provided with a pair of rubbers for use in each pen and a pan of disinfectant (a weak lysol solution) for dipping the soles of the shoes or rubbers before and after entering the pen or house. Visitors who have been handling poultry elsewhere should not enter the poultry house or yard.

Medicinal Agents and Their Use

While anthelmintic (worm-expelling) treatment has proved to be applicable to many kinds of livestock and has served to reduce parasitism in them to the point where it apparently does little or no harm, the use of medicinal agents in the control of poultry parasites has not met with any great success. Despite the large amount of experimental work done on the control of poultry parasites by means of medication, effective and practical drugs for the control of such economically important diseases as coccidiosis, blackhead and tapeworms are still lacking. Although some progress has been made in the treatment of other parasitic diseases of poultry, satisfactory drugs for the control of many of the roundworms are also lacking.

To be satisfactory, a drug designed for the removal of parasites from poultry must be inexpensive, relatively easy to administer, highly effective and relatively nontoxic, The value of the individual bird is ordinarily so low that the cost of administering drugs to fowls, unless mass treatment can be resorted to, is in most cases prohibitive.

Effective drugs have been discovered for the removal of the gapeworm, the large roundworm and the cecum worm and the treatment will be discussed briefly.

Hall and Shillinger (*17*) and others, have reported that carbon tetrachloride is an effective drug for the removal of the large intestinal roundworm, *Ascaridia galli*. Ackert and Graham (3) found carbon tetrachloride highly efficacious in removing the large intestinal roundworm from young chickens with apparently no ill effects.

For the control the cecum worm, Hall and Shillinger (*17*) recommend rectal injections of a mixture of oil of chenopodium and olive or cottonseed oil. McCulloch and Nicholson (*37*) stated that phenothiazine, given in either single or repeated doses, was very effective for the removal of cecum worms from chickens. Roberts (*40*) reported that phenothiazine was effective for the removal of the cecum worm but not of the large intestinal roundworm.

Wehr, Harwood and Schaffer (*53*) found that barium antimonyl tartrate given as an inhalant successfully removed a large percentage of the gapeworms (*Syngamus trachea*) from chicks, turkey poults and grown turkeys. For treatment, the infected birds are confined in a tight container into which the powder is introduced through an opening near the top by means of a dust gun (Fig. 1). The worms in the trachea are killed by the dust inhaled by the birds.

It has been demonstrated that trichomoniasis (infection with trichomonads) of the lower digestive tract of poultry can be successfully treated by means of heat therapy. Olsen and Allen (*38*) successfully treated a number of turkeys infected with *Trichomonas gallinarum* by placing them in a thermostatically controlled cabinet for periods ranging from 1 to 2 hours. The internal body temperature of the birds was raised from 2° to 6° above the normal temperature of 106.5° F. by maintaining an air temperature of approximately 104° F. and a relative humidity of 60 to 70 percent within the treatment box. These investigators found that three treatments at intervals of every

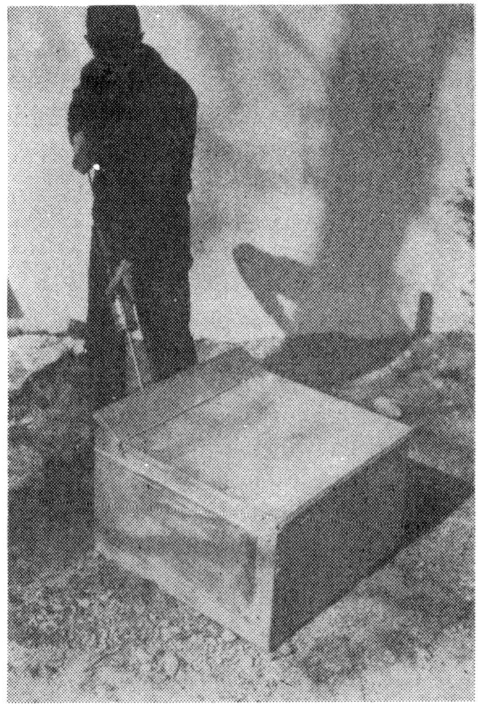

Fig. 1: Equipment for and method of administering barium antimonyl tartrate to chickens infected with gapeworms.

other day were sufficient to check the disease, but in advanced cases it was sometimes necessary to administer as many as six treatments. As soon as the body temperature returned to normal, the birds were removed from the cabinet and placed in wire-bottomed cages. Forced feeding of liquid mash was resorted to when the birds refused to eat voluntarily.

Occasionally a bird failed to respond to the heat treatment. Those that did respond usually began to eat voluntarily, gained in weight and behaved like normal, active birds after the second or third treatment. Several adult turkey hens were treated and later laid several clutches of eggs.

A few of the treated birds were killed at different stages of recovery following treatment and postmortem examinations disclosed that many of the liver lesions (tissue injuries) had almost completely disappeared and others were in the process of healing. Cultures made from partly healed lesions showed no trichomonads. A relatively large percentage of the untreated birds died from trichomoniasis.

No satisfactory treatment for trichomoniasis of the upper digestive tract has been developed.

The Protozoan Parasites of Poultry

The protozoan parasites of poultry that are significant as disease producers and therefore of concern to poultrymen belong to two major groups, the flagellates and the Sporozoa. The flagellates include actively moving protozoa equipped with from one to many whiplike hairs or flagella, which are used to propel the organism through the fluids in which they live. The Sporozoa, are spore-forming organisms, are almost exclusively parasitic and are characterized by the absence of definite organs for movement and by their peculiar, often complex life histories.

A species of the flagellated organisms scientifically designated as *Hexamita meleagridis* is suspected of playing an important role in the production of a severe intestinal infection in young turkeys known as infectious catarrhal enteritis (inflammation of the intestines). The part played by another flagellate, *Histomonas meleagridis,* in the production of so-called "blackhead" disease, or enterohepatitis (literally, inflammation of the intestines and the liver), of turkeys is well known. At least two species of flagellates of the genus *Trichomonas* are associated with intestinal disturbances of young turkeys, one producing caseating necrotic lesions (injuries characterized by the presence of cheesy matter and dead tissue) in the crop and esophagus, or gullet and the other responsible for large cecal (blindgut) and liver lesions similar in character to those of blackhead; these conditions have been designated as trichomoniasis of the upper digestive tract and of the lower digestive tract, respectively.

The most important sporozoan parasites of poultry are the coccidia, which are of such tremendous economic importance as the cause of coccidiosis in chickens that they are discussed in a separate article in this book. Two other sporozoan parasites that are arousing considerable attention and are believed to be responsible for, malaria like diseases of young ducks and turkeys are identified by most investigators as species of *Leucocytozoon.*

With the exception of the coccidia, the protozoan parasites of poultry have their greatest significance, from the disease standpoint, in turkeys. Other domestic birds such as chickens, ducks, geese, guinea fowl and pigeons frequently harbour similar or identical parasites, a few of which appear to be pathogenic, or disease-producing, to their hosts, while most are tolerated with little or no inconvenience. In the following discussion of specific diseases known or believed to be caused by protozoan parasites, primary emphasis is placed on turkeys, the host birds in which these disorders reach their largest proportions. The general principles of protozoan parasitism and parasite control, however, apply equally to other poultry.

Infectious Catarrhal Enteritis of Turkeys

Infectious catarrhal enteritis (hexamitiasis) of turkeys, associated with *Hexamita meleagridis,*[3] is becoming increasingly important in the United States. This disease has been known to exist in California for some time. It is apparently increasing in occurrence and severity with the expansion in turkey production, the increased crowding of birds on inches probably affording greater opportunities for turkeys to acquire the infection. The technical name "infectious catarrhal enteritis" indicates that the disease is a contagious intestinal inflammation characterized by abnormally heavy secretion from the mucous glands of the affected intestine.

Hexamitiasis is primarily an acute infection of the upper part of the small intestine of turkey poults between the ages of 1 and 12 weeks, with the greatest death loss occurring at 3 to 5 weeks of, age.

---

[3] Among other designations, the disease hits been described recently as a "trichomoniasis," but Hinshaw, McNeil, and Kofoid (*21*) presented convincing field and experimental evidence which definitely eliminated Trichomonas as the causative agent and implicated another protozoan parasite, a species of *Hexamita.* Hinshaw and McNeil (*20*) gave the specific name *meleagridis* to the *Hexamita* which they stated was "the causative agent of infectious catarrhal enteritis" in turkeys, In view of this recent information, there seems to be justification for designating the infection as hexamttiasis. The present discussion of the disease is based on the work of these investigators.

The symptoms of an acute outbreak are not very specific, being in general similar to those of other acute intestinal diseases. Sick poults are listless and droopy, walk with a stilted gait and often have a watery or foamy diarrhea. The birds may continue to eat but fail to digest and assimilate food normally, with rapid loss of flesh as a consequence. In individual birds, the acute infection runs a short. course of 1 to 6 days after symptoms appear, but in large flocks the peak of mortality during an outbreak occurs in 7 to 10 days after the irst sick birds are observed. Most birds that survive acute infections recover from the emaciation and remain stunted. Mortality icute outbreaks on California ranches has been reported to om 20 to 90 percent. Subacute infections sometimes occur, rized by listlessness and loss of weight in affected birds. ority of the birds that survive acute infections, as well as with subacute infections, become carriers and are potential irces of infection to young birds.

The chief sign of the disease seen on postmortem examination of birds that have died from acute hexamitiasis is catarrhal inflammation of the upper part of the small intestine. The intestinal contents are thin and abnormally watery. The intestinal walls have lost tone and may be thin and flabby, with local distended areas having an inflamed mucous membrane. *Hexamita meleagridis* may be consistently demonstrated under the microscope in scrapings from the affected intestinal wall and occurs in particularly large numbers in the inflamed distended areas. In severe cases the flagellates may occur throughout the entire small intestine. The enormous numbers of *Hexamita meleagridis* found in poults with enteritis have not been observed in healthy birds.

Hexamita meleagridis is a microscopic, spindle-shaped, flagellated protozoan measuring on the average about one twenty-five hundredth of an inch in length. It is readily distinguished in structure and movements from the trichomonads, which are often found associated with it in the cecal discharges of the same bird, by the absence of an undulating membrane along the edge of the body, by the absence of an axostyle, or "tail," at the hind end and by the fact that the *Hexamita* organism move rapidly in a fairly straight line rather than jerkily. This parasite reproduces by simple longitudinal splitting, each organism dividing frequently to form two individuals. In both diseased and carrier birds living flagellates are continually discharged in the droppings. Susceptible poults may acquire the infection by swallowing feed or soil contaminated with droppings containing the parasites.

Both field and experimental evidence point to *Hexamita meleagridis* as the sole or principal cause of catarrhal enteritis of turkey poults.

It has been definitely shown by investigators in California that the adult turkey is the primary source of infection. The causative agent of the disease has been transmitted to quail and from quail to turkeys. Field evidence indicates that quail may serve as an important carrier of the infection in some regions.

Histomoniasis, or So-called "Blackhead" Infection

Histomoniasis, or enterohepatitis, is an acute, highly fatal disease of turkeys attributed to infection with the protozoan parasite *Histomonas meleagridis*. Though the acute infection in chickens is usually mild and transitory, chickens have an important part in the complete picture of histomoniasis because they are established as carriers following primary infection and thus serve as a source of infection for susceptible turkeys. Since the principal sites of infection in diseased turkeys are the walls of the ceca and the liver, the disease is technically termed "infectious enterohepatitis," which indicates that it is a contagious infection involving the intestine and liver. Under farm conditions, histomoniasis probably includes most of the so-called blackhead of turkeys. Dark discolouration of the head is not a constant symptom of the disease, however and may be produced by disorders of the circulatory system due to other causes. It is therefore probably more appropriate to designate the disease as histomoniasis. The unfortunate nonspecific term blackhead might well be eliminated from the veterinary vocabulary. Although the technical name may seem difficult to laymen, usage would soon give it the same currepcy as such names as "coccidiosis" and "trichomoniasis."

Histomoniasis has forced the abandonment of turkey raising in many parts of this country. Application of the principles unearthed in recent researches, however, particularly those of Tyzzer and his associates, has again made turkey production a successful enterprise in these areas. Tyzzer's report (*45*) on histomoniasis summarized the detailed information on the modes of infection of susceptible birds and the form, structure and life history of the parasite that is the basis of the present conception of the disease.

Turkeys are susceptible to histomoniasis at any age up to maturity. The disease develops within 2 to 3 weeks after the susceptible birds acquire infective organisms by ingesting feed or soil contaminated with droppings from infected birds. The course of the disease is rapid, death usually occurring soon after the development of symptoms. Sick birds are weak, listless and droopy and usually have sulfur-coloured diarrhea. Dark discolouration of the head, as already noted, is not a constant symptom. Death may sometimes occur without visible symptoms. Histomoniasis in older birds is less acute than in young poults, the illness usually being more prolonged and the mortality lower. The great majority of the younger birds that develop the disease die, the mortality often being 100 percent.

On postmortem examination, birds dying from histomoniasis show greatly enlarged ceca, or blind pouches, that contain cheesy masses of tissue debris often infiltrated with blood. The cecal walls are thickened and congested and show large, ulcer-like lesions. The liver also usually appears somewhat enlarged and is blotched with characteristic, slightly sunken, reddish-gray lesions of various sizes. Thin sections from the cecal walls, when mounted on slides and stained appropriately for examination under the microscope, show *Histomonas* organisms among the surface cells lining the walls. The living parasites may often be recovered from the characteristic liver lesions and demonstrated under the microscope.

The histomonads are peculiar flagellated protozoa with certain amoeboid, or amoebalike, tendencies. As they occur in the cecal contents of carrier birds, they are normally more or less rounded bodies that usually show amoeboid movements of the protoplasm (that is, they are capable of pushing out temporary arms of protoplasm from their surfaces) as well as rhythmic rotatory movements produced by the beating of a single locomotor whip, or flagellum. They measure on an average about one two-thousandth of an inch in length, although individuals may be considerably larger and possess as many as four flagella.

Immediately upon establishment in the ceca of a susceptible host bird, the histomonads multiply rapidly, invade the mucous membrane of the cecal walls and become rounded tissue forms. Invasion of tissues is usually brief in the chicken, which recovers with only slight inconvenience, though deaths from histomoniasis among chickens have been known and typical cecal and liver lesions have been seen at autopsy. The histomonads usually persist in the cecal contents indefinitely and the chicken is established as a carrier of the infection. In the more susceptible turkey, invasion of tissues is so energetic that the histomonads gain access to the blood stream and are carried to the liver, where the characteristic lesions are produced. The infected birds usually die from severe cecal and liver infection (enterohepatitis). The few turkeys able to survive the acute infection also become carriers. Both chickens and turkeys with acute or carrier infections are sources of infection to new susceptible hosts, discharging living histomonads regularly in their droppings. When shed from infected birds, the histomonads are either free in the feces or housed in some manner not let clearly understood within the eggs of the cecal worm, *Heterakis gallinae*, which are also eliminated in the feces after being produced by the adult worms in the ceca of the host birds. New hosts acquire the infection by swallowing feed or soil contaminated with droppings containing the parasites, either free or within the eggs of the cecal worm.

Leucocytozoan Disease of Ducks and Turkeys

Turkey poults under 12 weeks of age and ducklings 10 days to a few weeks old are most susceptible to leucocytozoan disease. The general symptoms are common to both kinds of host birds and therefore the infections in the two need not be differentiated. In the young birds the disease strikes suddenly, with acute symptoms lasting only 2 or 3 days. Sick birds first lose appetite, become droopy and have a tendency to sit down from weakness or exhaustion. They seem to be thirsty and drink large amounts of water. Their breathing becomes heavy and they may crawl instead of walking. In the later stages of severe infections, the birds are excitable and when disturbed may fall over, lapse into a coma during which the breathing is laboured and die. Some very sick birds die after only a few minor convulsions. Blood removed from the vein of a bird sick with this condition shows greatly enlarged spindle-shaped cells, somewhat larger than the normal red blood cells, which contain the parasitic organisms. The most characteristic lesion at autopsy is an enlarged and blackened spleen. The birds that recover from acute infections may either remain permanently stunted or show no serious effects, but most become carriers of the infection. Mortality from the acute disease is reported to range from 0 to 100 percent in ducklings and from 10 to 50 percent in turkeys.

It was originally believed that the parasites invaded the white cells, or leucocytes, of the blood of infected birds and for this reason they were named *Leucocytozoon*. Some later investigators believed, however, that the red corpuscles rather than the leucocytes were the host cells. This question is still not settled definitely. Whatever these host cells may prove to be, they are greatly altered by parasitism with the leucocytozoa. The parasitized host cells become elongated to 4 or 5 times their normal length, with ends tapered to points. The full grown parasites, usually one to each host cell, are elongated, oval or bean-shaped structures that almost completely fill the parasitized cells exclusive of the tapered ends. The ultimate result of this parasitism is the destruction of the host cells, with anemia as a consequence. It has been suggested that the cause of the respiratory difficulties observed in birds with advanced, severe leucocytozoan disease may be due to mechanical blocking of the small capillaries of the lungs with these large parasites.

The large parasites inside the cells of the circulating blood of the host birds represent only a stage of the life history of *Leucocytozoon*. They develop further only when ingested by certain species of *Simulium*, or common blackflies, that feed on the blood of the infected birds. In the engorged blackflies, the leucocytozoa pass through a definite cycle of development and within a few days small infective forms known as sporozoites are present in the salivary glands. Some of these sporozoites are expelled into the blood stream of susceptible young birds on which the blackflies feed. In ducks, the sporozoites are said to penetrate the surface cells lining the small capillaries of the lungs, liver and spleen and to undergo generations of multiplication there that result in the production of enormous numbers of parasites. Eventually these products of multiplication are liberated into the blood stream and invade cells of the circulating blood, where they may be detected by means of stained blood smears. The entire life history has been determined to require only 2 to 3 days in the blackflies and 9 or 10 days in the host birds.[4]

Trichomoniasis of the Upper Digestive Tract of Turkeys

Trichomoniasis (that is, infection with trichomonads) of the upper digestive tract is characterized by the presence of peculiar

[4] Further details of research are given in citations *23*, *24*, *39*, *42*, and *48*.

cheesy lesions of dead tissues piled up to as high as approximately two-tenths of an inch above the surface of the mucous membranes of the esophagus and crop. The entire upper digestive tract is studded with small grayish-white nodules, or lumps, resembling the pustules found in nutritional roup. The mucous membrane is entirely destroyed, and an examination of the cheesy lesions or retained fluid of the upper digestive tract discloses countless numbers of flagellates. The lesions usually end abruptly at the zone dividing the esophagus from the proventriculus, or true stomach, indicating perhaps that the gastric juice of the true stomach may be detrimental to the survival of these organisms.

Sick birds are characterized by a depressed appearance, loss of appetite, sagging wings, emaciation and drooling at the mouth. The droppings are usually of the consistency of water and contain large numbers of the flagellated parasites. Young birds may die as soon as 1 day after the appearance of symptoms, but older birds may linger for several weeks. In older birds the region surrounding the crop usually appears depressed and sometimes pendulous. Although certain other diseases may produce similar symptoms birds that make repeated attempts to swallow, extend the head and neck and retain the crop fluid should be suspected of trichomoniasis. Often diagnosis can be confirmed by inspection of the mouths of sick birds, since the lesions frequently occupy visible portions of the upper digestive tract. Ordinarily mortality is slight, but it has been reported to range as high as 73 percent in nature flocks to 87 percent in young flocks.

Individuals of *Trichomonas gallinae* are roughly egg-shaped flagellates measuring on an average one twenty-five hundredth of an inch in length. They are extremely active trichomonads capable of rapid forward spiral locomotion produced by the beating of the flagella at the front end and movements of the protoplasmic flange, or undulating membrane, extending along the edge of the body. It is generally believed that these upper-digestive-tract trichomonads are distinct from those inhabiting the ceca and lower intestine of turkeys. They differ in certain aspects of structure and behaviour, in their respective sites of localization within the digestive tracts of the host birds and apparently in their disease-producing capabilities. As with the other protozoan infections of turkeys, a certain percentage of the adult birds become carriers of the trichomonads and thus serve as sources of infection to susceptible birds. Presumably infection of new hosts occurs through ingestion of contaminated feed, soil, or drinking water with living trichomonads discharged from infected birds either in the droppings or in the discharges from the mouth.[5]

Trichomoniasis of the Lower Digestive Tract of Turkeys

Turkeys are victims of another disease, which was believed by Allen (7) to be due to *Trichomonas gallinarum*, a flagellate commonly found in the ceca and lower intestine of chickens, turkeys, guinea fowl and probably other domestic fowls. Infection with these parasites is common in healthy chickens and turkeys, but disease symptoms develop with much greater frequency and severity in the latter. According to Allen (*8*) the infection resembles histomoniasis in producing lesions in the ceca and liver of turkeys, but these lesions are characteristically different from those of histomoniasis. The disease may be designated tentatively as "trichomoniasis of the lower digestive tract" to distinguish it from *T. gallinae* infection of the esophagus and crop.

Birds experimentally infected with *Trichomonas gallinarum* sometimes develop the acute type of infection, characterized by diarrhoea and occasional mortality in the young turkeys a few days after inoculation, but more often they develop a chronic type of the disease, the symptoms of which do not appear for several weeks after infection. Under certain conditions not yet fully understood, these trichomonads may produce an enterohepatitis, with lesions distinct from those of histomoniasis. Liver lesions have not been observed in experimentally or naturally infected birds under 3 months of age. The turkeys that develop the disease gradually and progressively lose their thrifty condition, become droopy, often have intermittent attacks of diarrhoea characterised by pale-yellow droppings and usually die. The slow, chronic development of the disease is sharply contrasted with the acuteness of histomoniasis. The importance of this type of trichomoniasis has not been fully determined. The insidious, chronic nature of the infection, its tendency to produce isolated loses rather than mass mortality and

---

[5] See citations 14, 19, 29, 32, 33, 43, 44, and 49 for further details of research.

the possible confusion of the specific lesions with those of histomoniasis have probably permitted the disease to go undetected. The studies of Allen indicate that it may prove to be of considerable importance.

The cecal and liver lesions are the most obvious changes to be observed at post mortem examination of birds dead of the disease. The liver lesions are the most clearly defined, being irregular, granular, often slightly elevated areas of cheesy appearance, quite distinct from the rounded, non-granular, noticeably depressed lesions of histomoniasis. Similar lesions are present on the cecal walls and often one or both ceca contain cores of cheesy, dead material infiltrated with blood. In naturally infected turkeys, the lesions may occur separately or together with those of histomoniasis and there appears to be basis for the belief that in the past the lesions of the two distinct diseases have often been collectively diagnosed as blackhead lesions. In the interest of accurate diagnosis and proper evaluation of their relative importance the two infections should be carefully differentiated.

Allen (7) expressed the opinion that the common cecal trichomonads of turkeys are identical with *Trichomonas gallinarum*, described previously from the chicken. These trichomonads are on an average considerably smaller but much more active than the histomonads, which may often occur in the same cecal contents from infected birds. They vary from nearly spherical to distinctly pear-shaped and their average length is approximately one thirty-five hundredth of an inch. They are typical trichomonads, each individual possessing several whips, or flagella and an undulating membrane along the edge of the body. The combined movements of these flagella and the undulating membrane give a jerky type of locomotion with little forward progression, characteristically different from the rapid forward, movements of *T. gallinae*.

As known at present, the life history of *Trichomonas gallinarum* is apparently simple. The trichomonads in the cecal contents of the host birds feed by absorption from the fluids in the lumen, or cavity, of the ceca and each individual periodically reproduces by asexual splitting to form two trichomonads. Infected birds regularly shed living trichomonads in the cecal droppings. No resistant, or cyst, forms have been observed in the course of the life history; and if no cysts are formed, it is evident that young birds must pick up living trichomonads very soon after they are discharged from infected birds, since these flagellates are extremely susceptible to drying and changes in temperature. Once ingested by susceptible birds in feed, soil, or drinking water, the parasites must survive the passage through the alimentary tract in order to become established in the lower intestine and ceca of the new host birds.

Metazoan Parasites of Poultry

Trematodes

Flukes, or trematodes, are small, flattened, unsegmented worms which as adults are parasites of both invertebrates and vertebrates. Most flukes are internal parasites, usually inhabiting the intestinal tract, lung, liver, or some other internal organ. A few, however, have been classified as external parasites, since they are found in the skin and similar locations.

At least three species of flukes have been reported as parasitizing poultry in the United States, but none of them is of any great economic importance. One species, *Collyriclum faba*, is an external parasite that occurs in the skin of domestic and wild birds. The other two species, *Prosthogonimus macrorchis* and *Psilostomum ondatrae*, are internal parasites, the former occurring in the bursa Fabricii (a glandular sac) and the egg-forming organs and the latter in the proventriculus.

The cystic or skin fluke, *Collyriclum faba*, has been reported from the domestic fowl in Minnesota and it has also been found in wild birds in Massachusetts, Maryland, Minnesota, Wisconsin, New Jersey, New York and Michigan.

These flukes produce small, hard, cyst-like structures, usually in the region of the vent. However, they have also been found in the skin just in front of the anus, in the chest region, over the lower surface of the abdomen and breast, around the beak on both the external and the internal surfaces, on the neck and on the crop.

The smooth, shiny, grayish-white cysts are one-twelfth to two-fifths inch (2 to 10 mm) in diameter and contain two approximately hemispherical flukes, in contact along their flattened surfaces. A dark-brown or almost black substance exudes from the opened cyst, which contains the minute eggs of the parasite.

The life history of the fluke is not completely known. It is believed that some snail is its first intermediate host and evidence points very definitely to nymphs of dragonflies as the second intermediate host. The eggs escape from the cysts through an opening in the cyst all and are scattered wherever the bird goes. Masses of degenerating and decaying cysts have been noted on chickens which, when they are removed or have dropped off, apparently serve to disseminate the disease, since the dead areas contain myriads of eggs. When brought into contact with water, the eggs hatch and apparently continue their development in a snail. The prevalence of this parasite in sparrows, crows, nuthatches and other land birds however, suggests that some land invertebrate may serve as the first intermediate host. Because of its prevalence in the English sparrow, it is thought that this bird may serve as an important disseminator of the disease.

The effects of the parasite on the fowl, aside from the possible slight injury to the general health of the bird and a disfigurement of the skin, which lowers the market value, are not noteworthy.

Proventriculitis (inflammation of the true stomach) in chickens may be due to a small fluke, *Psilostomum ondatrae*, commonly found in muskrats and water birds. The life history of this fluke is not known. The only report of the parasite's occurring in domestic fowl in the United States is from Colourado. Twenty-nine deaths in a flock of 42 White Leghorns 8 weeks old and, 8 deaths in a flock of Plymouth Rock pullets were attributed to infection with the parasite. Infected birds develop inappetence (lack of appetite) and lethargy and gradually waste away. After several days of sickness, death results, apparently from starvation. Post mortem findings are an enlarged and ulcerated proventriculus, a deep reddening around the openings of the glands, and, in severe cases of infection, a grayish exudate, or discharge, on the surface of the glandular stomach. The flukes apparently do not burrow into the proventriculus but produce the irritation by their presence on the surface of the mucous membrane.

A small, reddish-coloured fluke, nearly one-fourth of an inch long, occurs in the bursa Fabricii and oviduct of the domestic chicken and duck in the Great Lakes region. This parasite has been reported by Kotlan and Chandler (*30*) from the oviduct of a wing-pinioned duck in Michigan. Although believed by some investigators to be identical with *Prosthogonimus pellucidus*, a species of fluke occurring in a similar location in the domestic chicken and duck in Europe, this fluke has been described by Macy (*35*) as a new species, *P. macrorchis.*

Owing to its location within the reproductive organs, *Prosthogonimus macrorchis* may be responsible for serious losses, due to reduced or complete stoppage of egg production among laying hens. The symptoms shown by infected fowls are dullness, loss of weight and a greatly decreased egg production. Controlled experiments have shown that uninfected birds laid nearly 10 times as many eggs as the infected hens. In the oviduct, the parasites are responsible for acute inflammation and the formation of abnormal eggs. The irritation resulting from the presence of these flukes in the oviduct causes a reversal of the peristaltic movements, which results in broken yolks, albumen, bacteria and parasitic material entering the abdominal cavity and giving rise to acute peritonitis, or inflammation of the abdominal lining. Kotlan and Chandler (*30*) described the pathological changes resulting from the presence of these worms as–heavy emaciation and anaemia; fibrinous peritonitis, with a large amount of sticky, yellow exudate, containing large masses of egg-yolk and albumen material; a number of red-coloured., live flukes were found in the exudate. The ovary showed a number of diseased, collapsed ovules, containing grayish-yellow, egg-yolk-like material mixed with fibrin and pus. Some of the ovules were apparently ruptured. The oviduct was greatly distended, its serous coverings showing a more or less pronounced reddish discolouration. The lumen of the oviduct contained a large amount of albumen material forming ovoid clots of about one to two centimeters in diameter; the mucosa was covered with a sticky exudate consisting in the main of albumen, blood and fibrin.

The life cycle of the parasite involves two intermediate hosts, snails and dragonflies. Macy (*36*) found that the snail *Amnicola limosa porata,* which is common in the lakes of Michigan, Wisconsin, Minnesota and other Northern States, served as the first intermediate host. He succeeded in infecting dragonfly nymphs by placing a number of cercariae of *Prosthogonimus macrorchis* (the form of the organism found in snails) in Syracuse watch glasses containing the young dragonflies.

Kotlan and Chandler (*31*) demonstrated experimentally that chickens can become infected with the adult flukes by feeding them dragonfly nymphs containing cysts of *Prosthogonimus* species. It is believed that ducks are the normal hosts of *P. macrorchis* and the domestic hen is the abnormal host, as the latter loses its infection in 3 to 5 weeks. The rate of growth of the adult fluke is relatively slow in ducks and chicks but more rapid in the oviduct of the hen. The fluke develops only in the oviducts of laying hens and has been occasionally found in hen's eggs.

Cestodes

Tapeworms, or cestodes, are flattened or ribbon-shaped worms composed of numerous segments or divisions. The head, neck and a small number of the front segments are usually much narrower than the remaining portion of the worm, which grows from the neck backwards, so that the segments farthest removed from the head are the oldest from the standpoint of development. The terminal segments of the fully developed tapeworm may be filled with eggs; these are known as gravid segments and are the ones usually found in the droppings of infected birds.

Several species of tapeworms inhabit the small intestines of fowls. Each species usually shows some preference for a certain part of the small intestine to which to attach itself and develop. If tapeworms are present in large numbers, however, specimens may be found attached to portions of the intestine other than the one normally preferred.

So far as has been ascertained by experimentation, all poultry tapeworms pass the earlier part of their development in one of the lower animals. These so-called intermediate hosts include houseflies, snails, slugs, ants, earthworms; grasshoppers, sandhoppers and others.

Intermediate hosts become infected with young tapeworms by swallowing the gravid, or egg-bearing, segments which have been passed in the droppings of infected birds. Within the body cavity of the intermediate host, the bladder worm, or young tapeworm, has the appearance of a sac filled with liquid in the center of which is seen the head of the adult tapeworm. The head contains four cup-shaped cavities, or suckers and a number of hooks surround the front end.

When a susceptible bird host swallows an intermediate host containing these bladder worms, they attach themselves to the intestinal wall and begin to develop segments, which appear first just back of the head in the so-called neck or growing region.

The nodular tapewom, *Raillietina echinobothrida*, produces nodules or tuberclelike bodies in the subserous and muscular coats of the walls of the posterior (hind) portion of the small intestines of chickens and other fowls. These lesions closely resemble those of, avian tuberculosis and it is important that a careful examination be made before a positive diagnosis is given. The diagnosis should not be difficult, since nodules in the wall of the small intestine in the absence of tapeworms may be considered as being due to the tubercle bacillus and not to the nodular tapeworm. The tapeworm may be quite small and may be overlooked in a hurried or cursory examination. In case of doubt, the affected intestine should be opened and washed carefully in a stream of water. The washed intestine is then placed in a dish of water deep enough to cover it; if tapeworms are present, they will be seen hanging to the mucous membrane. This discovery, in the absence of lesions in the liver or other organs, would warrant the diagnosis of tapeworm disease.

Jones and Horsfall (*26, 27*) showed that the ants *Tetramorium caespitum* and *Pheidole vinelandica* naturally harboured bladder worms of this tapeworm and also those of another closely related species, *Raillietina tetragona*. When these two bladder worms were fed to young chickens, the latter became infected with the adults of the cestodes. Joyeux and Baer (*28*) reported finding bladder worms of *R. echinobothrida* in naturally infected ants, *Tetramorium semilaeve*, in the region of Marseilles, France.

The proliferating, or branching, tapeworm, *Hymenolepis cantaniana*, occurs in the small intestines of chickens, quail, pheasants, turkeys and peafowl.

Alicata and Jones (*6*) found that the small dung beetle, *Ataenius cognatus*, served as an intermediate host of this tapeworm. As found in the infected beetle, the young tapeworm consists of numerous branches with a few terminal buds which represent completely developed bladder worms. From 2 to 3 weeks are required for the bladder worm to develop into the adult tapeworm in the avian host.

The broad-headed tapeworm, *Raillietina cesticillus*, attaches itself by preference to the anterior (front) and middle portions of the small intestine of the chicken, guinea fowl and turkey. This tapeworm is probably one of the most common cestodes of domestic fowls in the United States. It may be readily distinguished from other species of tapeworms infecting poultry by the broadly developed head, which carries a double row of 400 to 500 delicate, hammer-shaped hooks; the suckers are weakly developed and devoid of spines.

Several species of beetles belonging to the families Scarabaeidae, Tenebrionidae and Carabidae have been shown experimentally to serve as intermediate hosts for *Raillietina cesticillus*. The meal beetles, *Tribolium castaneum* and *T. confusum*, which are commonly found infesting poultry feeds, have been shown recently to serve in this capacity.

Ackert and Reid (*4*) demonstrated experimentally that chiekens 2½ to 5 months of age are more resistant to infection with this species of tapeworm than younger birds and that a reduction in the blood sugar and haemoglobin contents of the blood resulted from such infections. Harwood and Luttermoser (*18*) reported that the growth of Rhode Island Red and White Leghorn chicks was retarded by infections with the tapeworm.

The minute tapeworm *Davainea proglottina* usually inhabits the duodenal region (the first part of the small intestine) of the chicken, turkey and occasionally other birds. In heavy infections, individual tapeworms may be found as far back as the yolk stalk. This tapeworm has been reported from widely separated areas in the United States, but most often from the Eastern States. It is one of the smallest tapeworms found infecting poultry. A fully developed specimen measures about one-fiftieth to three twenty-fifths of an inch in length and is composed of two to five segments which gradually increase in length and breadth as the worm matures; the last segment may be larger than all the rest of the parasite. Because of its small size, this tapeworm is frequently overlooked.

The life cycle of *Davainea proglottina* was first demonstrated experimentally by Grassi and Rovelli (*15*) who showed that the common garden slug, also called the gray field slug, *Agriolimax agrestis*, could be successfully infected with the bladder worms of this tapeworm. In addition to this slug, many other species of slugs and two species of snails, *Polygyra thyroides* and *Zonitoides arboreus*, have been incriminated experimentally as intermediate hosts of the tapeworm. The gray field slug is very common in those sections from which *D. proglottina* has been reported and probably plays a very important role in the perpetuation of the disease wherever it and the parasite occur together.

This species has been considered by a number of investigators to be one of the obviously dangerous tapeworms infecting poultry. Heavily infected birds are said to become lethargic and waste away. On post mortem examination the intestinal mucous membrane appears thickened, which may be due to haemorrhages and the intestine contains a large quantity of mucus, which tends to be fetid. Leg weakness has been attributed to infections with this tapeworm, but its true relationship to this condition is still unknown.

Domesticated fowls are hosts of a number of other species of tapeworms. *Hymenolepis carioca* is a very common cestode of poultry in the United States. It is a small tapeworm measuring 1⅕ to 3⅛ inches long, threadlike and very fragile; the segments break off easily when handled. It sometimes occurs in large numbers in chickens and turkeys, but it has very little, if any, effect on the growth rate of young chicks. This species of tapeworm utilizes the dung beetles, *Onthophagus hecate, Aphodius granarius, Choeridium histeroides* and others as intermediate hosts.

Metroliasthes lucida, a common cestode of turkeys, measures as much as 8 inches (20 cm) in length. It lacks a rostellum (beak) and the suckers are devoid of spines. Jones (25) found that the eggs of this tapeworm would develop to the bladderworm stage in grasshoppers.

Amoebotaenia sphenoides is principally a parasite of chickens. This tapeworm measures only from one-twelfth to one-sixth inch (2 to 4 mm) long; the head has a single row of 14 hooks and is followed by a short neck. The 18 to 20 segments that follow the neck gradually increase in size up to the fourteenth and then gradually decrease. It has been demonstrated that a species of earthworm, *Ocnerodrilus africanus*, served as an intermediate host of this tapeworm. More recently, the earthworms *Helodrilus foetidus, Pheretina pequana* and *Allolobrophora chloritica* have been assigned to this role. Chickens in Texas, Kansas and Michigan have been reported as being infected with this species of tapeworm.

Under normal conditions this parasite probably causes very little damage to fowls.

Choanotaenia infundibulum, a cestode parasite of the duodenum, or forward part of the small intestine, of chickens, turkeys, and, several species of wild game birds, is frequently met within chickens and turkeys in the United States. Houseflies, grasshoppers and several species of beetles have been reported as intermediate hosts of this tapeworm.

Nematodes

Roundworms, or nematodes, are usually elongated, cylindrical, unsegmented worms which vary from only a small fraction of an inch to several inches in length. They likewise differ greatly in habitat, having been found in poultry in almost every organ.

On the basis of their life histories, the roundworms of poultry may be divided into two general groups:

(1) Those transmitted directly from bird host to bird host, and

(2) those requiring an insect, or some other lower animal for their complete development.

The first type of life cycle is considered the simplest, for its completion involves merely the swallowing by a host animal of the embryonated roundworm eggs (those containing embryos, which are infective) with the food and water or bits of soil. The embryo roundworm hatches in the intestinal tract and direct development to the adult stage usually takes place there. Soon after hatching, the young of many of the species of roundworms of poultry penetrate into the mucosa, or lining of the intestinal tract and usually spend a number of days there before re-entering the intestinal cavity. In the case of the gapeworm, the young worms leave the alimentary tract and wander through various organs of the body before settling down permanently in the trachea, or windpipe.

In addition to the roundworms that pass part of their development in insects or some other form of animal life, thus requiring a true intermediate host, a third group is recognized in which the infective stage is transmitted either directly, through the medium of contaminated food and water, or indirectly, by swallowing some insect or other animal in the body of which the infective stage has encysted. The gapeworm of poultry is an example of the latter group.

Crop Worms

Domestic fowls are susceptible to infection with at least three species of crop worms, namely, *Capillaria annulata*, *C. contorta* and *Gongylonemia ingluvicola*. The first two species. are commonly known as capillarid worms, threadworms, or hairworms, while the last has been called the gullet worm.

These crop worms are long and slender, varying in length from half an inch to 2 or more inches. They bury themselves in the mucous membrane of the crop and esophagus, or gullet, in tortuous burrows, from which it is often difficult to remove them whole (Fig. 2). In heavy infections, these worms may be found in the undilated portion of the esophagus as well as the dilated portion or crop.[6]

The life histories of the two threadworms are known, but that of the gullet worm is yet to be discovered. The transmission of *Capillaria contorta* was found to be direct by Cram (*12*). At about the same time (1936) Wehr (*50*) discovered that *Capillaria annulata* required the earthworm as all intermediate host.

The chief injury produced by the crop worms is a thickening of the wall and an enlargement of the glands of the crop and esophagus. In heavy infections the crop wall is greatly thickened, highly inflamed and congested and the mucous membrane is loose and torn.

Stomach Worms

The proventriculus, or true stomach, is the site of infection by two parasitic roundworms, *Dispharynx spiralis* and *Tetrameres americana.*

The spiral stomach worm, *Dispharynx spiralis,* has been observed in the proventriculus of the chicken, turkey, guinea fowl, pigeon and a few wild gallinaceous birds (the same order to which domestic poultry belong). In certain sections of the United States, particularly

[6] Wehr (*51*) observed that each of these three species of roundworms, when viewed in their normal position in the mucosa of the esophagus, displayed a different body contour. This discovery afforded a reasonably accurate method of identifying the worms at the site of the infection without resorting to a detailed microscopic examination of each worm. All three species assume a twisted position in the mucosa, but in the case of the gullet worm the perspective is one of a series of folds approximately uniform in size and shape, following one another in close succession and usually extending in a straight course. In the two species of Capillaria, the body shape consists of a series of irregularly shaped folds. However, *Capillaria annulata* may be readily distinguished from *Capillaria contorta* by its much smaller size. In case of doubt the particular worm may be removed from its burrow and examined microscopically for the presence of a cuticular swelling directly back of the head which identifies it as *Capillaria annulata.*

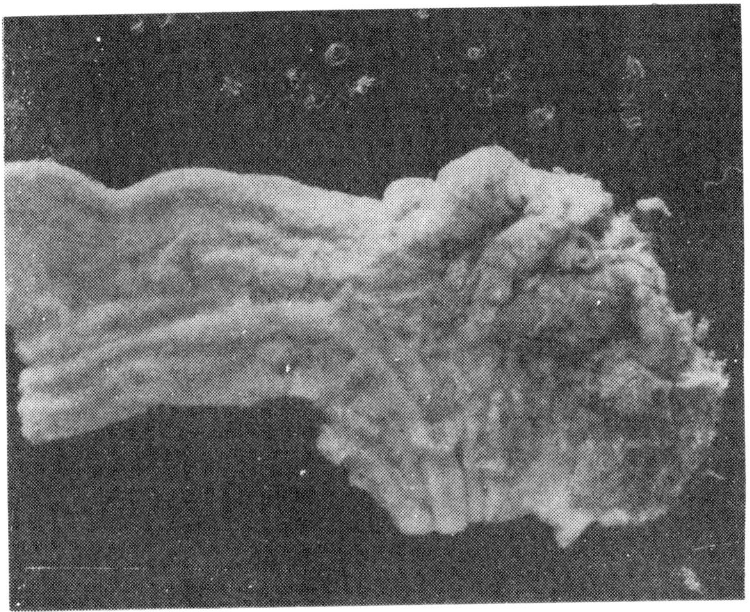

Fig. 2: Crop and esophagus of a bird heavily infested with the crop worm, *Capillaria annulata.*

California and Texas, pigeons have been found to be very heavily infected with this parasitic roundworm.

The adult worms are short and thick and usually are curved or rolled in the form of a spiral; the hind end of the male is very tightly coiled. At the site of infection, the nematodes are usually found with their heads buried deeply in the wall of the proventriculus. Tumors are usually formed at the site of the attachment of the worms and in heavy infections the wall of the glandular, or true, stomach becomes enormously and uniformly thickened as well as ulcerated.

Cram demonstrated experimentally that the pill bug serves as the intermediate host of the spiral stomach worm. Whether it is the principal intermediate host for the spread of the parasite under natural conditions is not known.

The globular roundworm, *Tetrameres americana*, is strikingly different in appearance from most roundworms. The male worm is very small and in general resembles other nematodes, but the female is globular and bright red. The two sexes likewise differ in their location within the stomach. The female worms, apparently when quite young, enter the tubular glands (Lieberkiuhn's glands) of the stomach wall, leaving only the hind part of the body, including the vulva, protruding into the stomach cavity. The male lives free in the cavity of the stomach and apparently enters Lieberkuhn's glands only for a short time to mate with the female.

Infective larvae of *Tetrameres americana* have been recovered from the body cavities of the grasshoppers *Melanoplus femur-rubrum* and *M. differentialis* 42 days after experimental infection. Chickens to which infected grasshoppers were fed later became infected with the adults of this stomach worm. Barber (9) stated that *T. americana* was the cause of a serious catarrhal condition in chickens in Guam. In heavy infections the walls of the proventriculus become so swollen that the cavity is almost obliterated.

Gizzard Worms

Of the parasitic roundworms occurring underneath the thick, horny lining of the gizzard of poultry, only two species are of economic importance. These worms burrow through the horny lining of the gizzard and bury themselves, sometimes deeply, in the muscles beneath. The gizzard worm of chickens and turkeys, *Cheilospirura hamulosa*, selects the anterior and posterior (front and back) portions of the gizzard, regions in which the horny covering is thin and soft, while the gizzard worm of ducks and geese, *Amidostomum anseris*, maybe found generally throughout this organ.

In life these worms are reddish in colour, indicating perhaps that they are bloodsuckers. The damage they cause to the gizzard may be so severe that this organ cannot function properly; thus they interfere with the digestion of the bird.

Cheilospirura hamulosa requires an intermediate host for its complete development. Several species of grasshoppers and numerous beetles, including the common meal beetle, *Tribolium castaneum*, have been found experimentally to serve in this capacity.

In lightly infected birds the lining of the gizzard may show a slight ulcerative condition, which may involve the muscular tissue as well. Soft nodules inclosing the nematodes are sometimes found in the muscular portion of the gizzard, especially in the thinner parts. In heavy infections a large part of the posterior portion of the gizzard may become enlarged and frequently loses its natural shape. The symptoms vary with the degree of infection. Mild infections are scarcely detectable, whereas severe ones are said to produce anemia and emaciation.

Amidostomum anseris frequently occurs underneath the horny lining of the gizzard of ducks and geese, sometimes in large numbers. Cram (*11*) reported a severe outbreak of this disease among a flock of geese in New York. The owner of the flock reported a large number of deaths as a result of the outbreak.

The life history of this nematode is direct. The eggs are voided in the droppings and readily hatch in the presence of moisture. The newly hatched larvae reach the infective stage within a few days; when picked up by a susceptible host, the infective larvae develop to the adult stage in the gizzard.

Young infected birds show symptoms of dullness, loss of appetite and emaciation. The clinical symptoms are largely the result of the improper functioning of the diseased gizzard. On post mortem examination, the inner surfaces of the gizzard, in cases of heavy, infections, appear necrotic, or characterized by dead tissue; the heavy lining is loosened or sloughed in places and appears dark brown or black at the site of infection.

Large Intestinal Roundworms

One of the commonest and perhaps the most frequently seen of the parasitic roundworms of poultry is the large intestinal roundworm of chickens, *Ascaridia galli*. This parasite is very common wherever chickens are raised. It has occasionally been found in turkeys and its occurrence in ducks and geese has been reported. Similar worms, *Ascaridia columbae* and *Ascaridia numidae*, are frequently found in considerable numbers in the intestines of pigeons and guinea fowl, respectively.

The mature worms of the three species named range in length from 1½ to 4 inches. The chicken worm is the longest and slenderest, averaging in thickness about the size of the lead of an ordinary pencil. Specimens of this ascarid have been removed on a number of occasions from broken eggs. The worms had presumably wandered up the oviduct from the intestine via the cloaca and were later incorporated in the developing egg.

The life histories of two of these ascarids have been worked out and found to be similar. Since the life history of *Ascaridia galli* (Fig. 3) has been more fully discussed in the scientific literature than the others, it will be only briefly reviewed here. The eggs are deposited by the female in the cavity of the intestinal tract and pass out in the droppings of the infected bird. Before these eggs become infective, they must remain outside the body of the bird host at least 2 to 3 weeks. Susceptible birds become infected by ingesting food or water

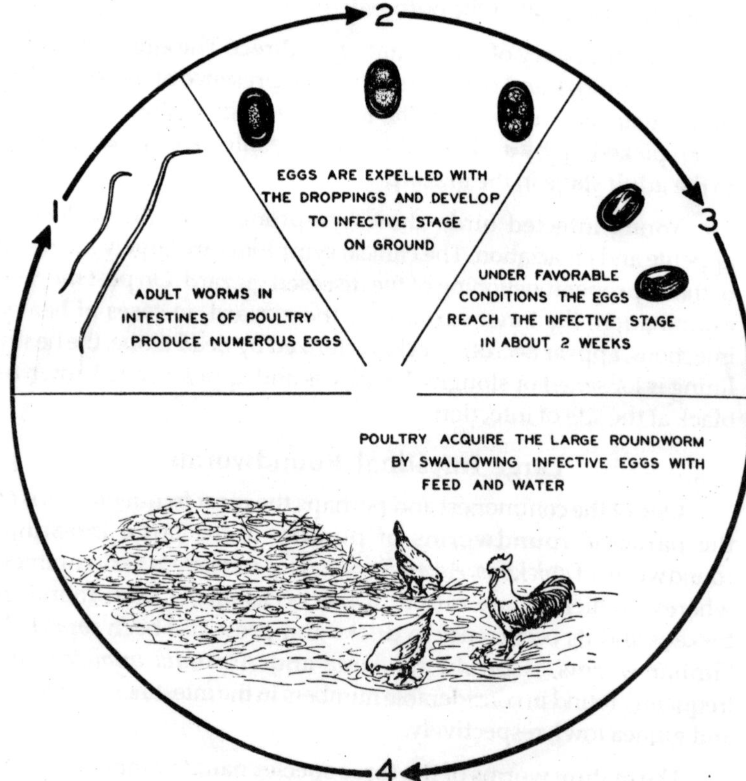

Fig. 3: Life-history chart of the large roundworm of the chicken, *Ascaridia galli*.

containing the infective eggs. According to Itagaki (22), the infective eggs hatch either in the proventriculus or the duodenum. Ackert (1) observed that the young worms lived free in the cavity of the posterior portion of the duodenum for the first 9 days, after which they penetrated the intestinal mucous membrane and caused hemorrhages (Fig. 4). By the seventeenth or eighteenth day, the young worms have left the mucous membrane and thereafter are to be found free in the cavity of the duodenum. Maturity is reached in about 50 days.

Chickens 3 to 4 months of age or older are quite resistant to parasitism with *Ascaridia galli.* Ackert, Edgar and Frick (2) stated that a relationship existed between the number of duodenal goblet cells (goblet-shaped cells on the membrane) and the mucin (the principal protoplasm in mucus) which these cells secreted and the development of the natural resistance of the growing chickens to

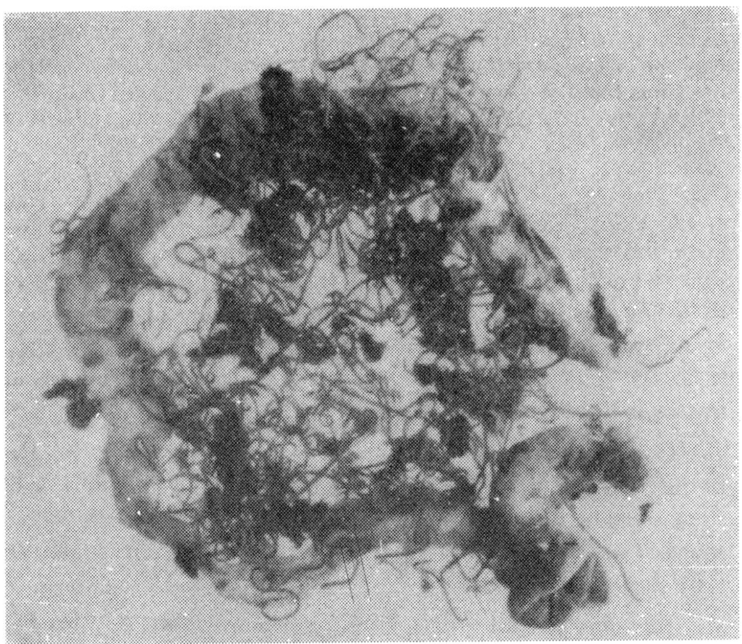

Fig. 4: Portion of the intestine of a bird, slit open to show the large number of roundworms.

this nematode. Since more goblet cells per area were found in the epithelial, or surface, lining of the duodenum of chickens 4 months old than in younger birds, the authors concluded that these cells were in some way responsible for the greater resistance developed by the older birds. The age at which the peak of the goblet-cell formation occurred was found to correspond very closely to the development of the maximum resistance of the chicken to the growth of the nematodes.

Animal proteins in the form of milk and meat have been shown to be important dietary supplements in the development of resistance of chickens to *Ascaridia galli* and a diet wholly of plant origin was not found to be conducive to resistance to helminth (worm) invasion. Ackert and his co-workers have shown that foods high in vitamins A and B increase the fowl's resistance to this nematode and that the lack of the vitamin B complex definitely favors parasitism.

Birds heavily infected with *Ascaridia galli* have been found to suffer from loss of blood, reduced blood-sugar content, increased urates, shrunken thymus glands and retarded growth and mortality among them greatly increased. Droopiness, emaciation and diarrhea are symptoms of a heavily parasitized condition. Death sometimes results if treatment is not given.

Small Intestinal Roundworms

Several species of hairworms, or capillarids (*Capillaria* species), occur in the small intestines and ceca of domestic fowls. Since these worms are small and hairlike in appearance and from one-half to three-fourths of an inch long, they may be easily overlooked on a casual examination of the opened intestine at autopsy. It is, therefore, necessary to resort to the microscope to make sure of their presence in case of light infections.

One species, *Capillaria columbae,* has commonly been observed in the intestines of pigeons and less commonly in the intestines of the mourning dove, chicken and turkey. Uninfected birds become infected with this roundworm by swallowing the embryonated egg with the food and water.

Birds heavily infected with this hairworm show symptoms of emaciation, listlessness and diarrhea. Such birds spend much of their time in a huddled position on the ground. Their feathers are ruffled and soiled around the vent and the skin and visible mucous membranes are more or less pale. Food and water are taken sparingly. Death may occur as a result of heavy infections.

Leville (*34*) reported that the intestines of chickens heavily infected with *Capillaria columbae* under experimental conditions showed a moderate thickening of the mucous membrane, which contained "reddish areas varying from pinhead hemorrhagic spots to diffuse hyperemia (excess of blood) of large portions of the mucosa." The writer has observed that the intestines of heavily infected pigeons showed extensive destruction of the mucous membrane, which was frequently completely sloughed off and contained a large quantity of fluid.

The roundworm *Ornithostrongylus quadriradiatus* may be the cause of serious intestinal disturbances in pigeons. Turtledoves and mourning doves have also been reported as hosts. The eggs of this roundworm are voided in the droppings and hatch within 19 to 24 hours. Three to four days more are required for the young larvae to become infective. When the infective larvae are swallowed by a pigeon or other susceptible host, they mature in the small intestines and the female worms begin to deposit eggs 5 or 6 days after the larvae are ingested.

Cuvillier (*19*) reported that heavily parasitized birds become droopy and have ruffled feathers, with head and neck retracted. The birds remain squatting on the ground; if disturbed, they try to move but usually tip forward on the breast and head. Food is taken sparingly and is frequently regurgitated, along with bile-stained fluid. The birds usual drink an excessive amount of water. There is a pronounced greenish diarrhea and the birds lose weight rapidly. Death is preceded by prostration and difficult, rapid breathing. The intestines of fatally infected birds are markedly haemorrhagic and have a green mucoid content, with masses of cast-off membrane tissue.

The cecum worm of poultry, *Heterakis gallinae*, occurs commonly in the ceca of chickens, turkeys and possibly other domestic fowls. This worm attains a length of three-tenths to one-half inch. The life history is direct. The embryonated eggs hatch in the upper part of the intestine and at the end of 24 hours the majority of the young worms have reached the ceca.

The chief economic importance of the cecum worm lies in its role as a carrier of the causative agent of blackhead. Graybill and

Smith (*16*) discovered that blackhead can be produced by feeding large numbers of embryonated eggs of *Heterakis gallinae* removed from blackhead-infected birds. They offered the tentative hypothesis that the worms lowered the resistance of the host to the causative parasites already present in the ceca. Tyzzer and Fabyan (*47*), however, presented evidence which indicated that the protozoan parasite is incorporated in the worm egg, but they were unable to demonstrate its presence there.

Two other species of cecum worms, *Heterakis beramporia* and *H. eisolonche*, produce nodules in the ceca of chickens and pheasants, respectively.

Studies by Alicata (*5*) in Hawaii have shown that various insects, such as beetles and earwigs, serve experimentally as intermediate hosts of *Subulura brumpti*, a common pinworm of the ceca of chickens in the Hawaiian Islands.

An extremely small roundworm, *Strongyloides avium*, has been found in the ceca and small intestine of chickens in Louisiana and Puerto Rico. The walls of the ceca and small intestine of infected birds may be greatly thickened and a bloody diarrhea may be present. If infected chicks survive the acute stage, they may, when fully grown, show no in effects from the parasite, even though it is present. Young chickens may die as a result of a heavy infection, but if the infection is very light little or no clinical effect has been noted.

The life history of this nematode is direct. The eggs pass out of the fowl's body in the droppings. They hatch within 18 to 24 hours and the young worms develop in the soil into adult males and females, which shortly give rise to other young. These feed, molt and in turn either develop into adult males and females or transform to another type of larvae known as infective larvae. When these infective larvae are swallowed by a susceptible host, infection results. Unlike most species of nematodes, the parasitic cycle of *Strongyloides avium* consists of females only.

The Eye Worm

The eye worm of poultry, *Oxyspirura mansoni* is found only in Florida and Louisiana. The white worms are round beneath the nictitating membrane, or third eyelid, sometimes in large numbers.

Studies by Sanders (*41*) in Florida showed that the cockroach *Leucophala surinamensis* is the intermediate host of the chicken eye worm. The eggs of the female worms are washed down the tear ducts, swallowed and pass to the exterior in the droppings. The cockroach ingests the eggs or newly hatched larvae and the latter develop to the infective stage in the body cavity of the insect. When the cockroach is subsequently eaten by a chicken or other susceptible host, the infective larva is freed in the crop and passes up the esophagus to the mouth and then through the nasolachrymal duct (the tear duct) to the eye. Affected birds show signs of uneasiness and scratch at the eyes, which exhibit an acute inflammation accompanied by an abundant secretion of tears. The nictitating membrane is swollen, projects slightly beyond the eyelids at the corners of the eye and is kept in continual motion as if to remove Some foreign body from the eye. The eyelids sometimes become stuck together and a white cheesy matter collects beneath them. Occasionally severe ophthalmia (inflammation of the eye) develops and the eyeball may be destroyed if treatment of some sort is not resorted to. When this stage is reached the worms are no longer to be found in the eye. Severely affected birds eat very little, decline in strength, become anemic and may die within a few weeks.

Gapeworm

Gapeworm infection, commonly known as gapes, is caused by roundworms that live in the windpipe. These worms, *Syngamus trachea*, are sometimes called red worms because of their red colour or forked worms because the males and females so firmly adhere to one another that they appear like the letter **Y**. The male worm attains a length of about one-fifth of an inch, while the female reaches a length of nearly 1 inch.

This parasite has a direct life history. Eggs are coughed up from the windpipe and swallowed by the bird. They pass out in the droppings and develop and some of them hatch. Fowls become infected by swallowing either the infective eggs or the young roundworms that hatch from them. Earthworms may swallow the infective eggs or the young roundworms and are then a source of infection to fowls that swallow them.

The worms clog the windpipe of young poultry, causing them to sneeze, cough and gape for air (Fig. 5). An extensive irritation of the mucous lining of the windpipe results from the, bloodsucking activities of the gapeworms and coughing is apparently caused by this irritation. Similar symptoms result from brocchitis and

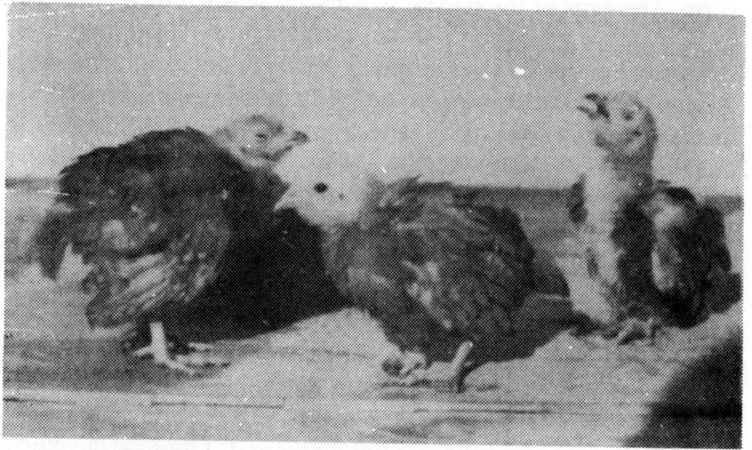

Fig. 5: Young chickens infected with gapeworms. The chicken on the right is gaping as a result of obstruction of the trachea by the worms.

laryngotracheitis, but if gapeworms are responsible they can be readily found by destroying a sick bird and slitting open the windpipe. The red, Y-shaped worms, if present, are usually found in the lower half of the windpipe.

Lesions or nodules are usually found at the point of attachment of the male worms only. Hence, it is believed that the male worm usually remains permanently attached to the tracheal wall, while the female worm loosens her hold from time to time and selects a new feeding place. Nodule formation occurs frequently in the tracheas of infected turkeys but is rarely seen in infected chicks because the latter rarely remain infected long enough for it to take place.

Affected birds become weak and emaciated and spend much of their time huddled on the floor with the eyes closed and the head drawn back against the body. The head is regularly thrown forward and upward and the mouth is opened wide to draw in air, or the head may be given a convulsive shake in an attempt to chosen the obstruction in the windpipe, so that normal breathing may be resumed. Sudden death is due primarily to suffocation caused by the mechanical obstruction of the windpipe by the rapidly growing worms and the accumulation of secreted mucus.

Wehr (52) observed that young turkey poults usually develop gapeworm symptoms in approximately 7 or 8 days, whereas young chickens do not ordinarily show symptoms of gaping and coughing until 10 to 14 days after experimental infection. The turkey poults likewise begin to die from gapeworm infections sooner than young chickens. Characteristic gapeworm symptoms of coughing and gaping have not been observed in guinea fowl and ducks. Young pheasants, however, suffer from the disease to an extent comparable, to that of young chicks and turkey poults. Older birds, unless heavily infected, usually show only mild symptoms or none at all. Chickens more than 10 weeks of age seldom harbour gapeworms under natural conditions. It has been reported, however, that in Ceylon gapeworms occur commonly in fowls of all ages, even up to 3 years. The role played by wild birds in the spread of gapeworm disease is still questionable.

Literature Cited

(1) ACKERT, JAMES E. (1931). THE MORPHOLOGY AND LIFE HISTORY OF THE FOWL NEMATODE ASCARIDIA LINEATA (SOHNEIDER). Parasitology 23: 360-379, illus.

(2) _____EDGAR, S.A. and FRICK, L.P. (1939). GOBLET CELLS AND AGE RESISTANCE OF ANIMALS TO PARASITISM. Amer. Micros. Soc. Trans. 58: 81-89.

(3) _____and GRAHAM, G.L. (1935). THE EFFICACY OF CARBON TETRACHLORIDE IN ROUNDWORM CONTROL. Poultry Sci. 14: 228-281, illus.

(4) _____and REID, W.M. (1937). AGE RESISTANCE OF CHICKENS TO THE CESTODE RAILLIETINA CESTICILLUS (MOLIN). (Abstract) Jour. Parasitol, 23: 558.

(5) ALICATA, JOSEPH E. (1939). PRELIMINARY NOTE ON THE LIFE HISTORY OF SUBULURA BRUMPTI, A COMMON CECAL NEMATODE OF POULTRY IN HAWAII. (Research note) Jour. Parasitol. 25: 179-180, illus.

(6) _____and JONES, MYRNA F. (1933). THE DUNG BEETLE, ATAENIUS COGNATUS, AS THE INTERMEDIATE HOST OF HYMENOLEPIS CANTANIANA. (Abstract of paper) Jour. Parasitol. 19: 244, illus.

(7) ALLEN, ENA A. (1940). A REDESCRIPTION OF TRICHOMONAS GALLINARUM MARTIN AND ROBERTSON, 1911, FROM THE CHICKEN AND TURKEY. Helminthol. Soc. Wash. Proc. 7: 65-68, illus.

(8) _____(1941). MACROSCOPIC DIFFERENTIATION OF LESIONS OF HISTOMONIASIS AND TRICHOMONIASIS IN TURKEYS. Amer. Jour. Vet. Res. 2:214-217, illus.

(9) BARBER, L.B. (1916). LIVE STOCK DISEASE INVESTIGATIONS. Guam Agr. Expt. Sta. Rpt. 1915: 25-41, illus.

(10) BISHOPP, F.C. (1927). THE FOWL TICK AND HOW PREMISES MAY BE FREED FROM IT. U.S. Dept. Agr. Farmers' Bul. 1070, 14pp., illus. (Revised.)

(11) CRAM, ELOISE B. (1926). A PARASITIC NEMATODE AS THE CAUSE OF LOSSES AMONG DOMESTIC GEESE. North Amer. Vet. 7. 27-29, illus.

(12) _____(1936). SPECIES OF CAPILIARIA PARASITIC IN THE UPPER DIGESTIVE TRACT BIRDS. U.S. Dept. Agr. Tech. Bull. 516, 28 pp., illus.

(13) CUVILLIER, EUGENIA (1937). THE NEMATODE, ORNITHOSTRONGYLUS QUADRIRADIATUS, A PARASITE OF THE DOMESTICATED PIGEON. U.S. Dept Agr. Tech. Bull. 569, 36 pp., illus.

(14) GIERKE, A.G. (1933). TRICHOMONIASIS OF THE UPPER DIGESTIVE TRACT OF CHICKENS. Calif. Dept. Agr., Monthly Bull. 22; 205-208, illus.

(15) GRASSI, B. and ROVELLI, G. (1888). DEVELOPMENT EXPERIMENTAL DU TAENIA PROGLOTTINA DAV. (Revue) Rec. de Med. vet. 65: 675-676.

(16) GRAYBILL, H.W. and SMITH THEOBALD (1920). PRODUCTION OF FATAL BLACKHEAD IN TURKEYS BY FEEDING EMBRYONATED EGGS OF HETERAKIS PAPILIOSA. Jour. Expt. Med. 31. 647-655.

(17) HALL, MAURICE C. and SHILLINGER, JACOB E. (1923). MISCELLANEOUS TESTS OF CARBON TETRACHLORIDE AS AN ANTHELMINTIC. Jour. Agr. Res. 23; 163-192.

(18) HARWOOD, PAUL D. and LUTTERMOSER, GEORGE W. (1938). THE INFLUENCE OF INFECTIONS WITH THE TAPEWORM, RAILLETINA CESTICILLUS, ON THE GROWTH OF CHICKENS. Helminthol. Soc. Wash. Proc. 5: 60-62.

(19) HAWN, M.C. (1937). TRICHOMONIASIS OF TURKEYS. Jour. Infect. Dis. 61; [184]-197.

(20) HINSHAW, W.R. and McNEIL, E. (1941). CARRIERS OF HEXAMITA MELEAGRIDIS. Amer. Jour. Vet. Res. 2: 453-458.

(21) _____McNEIL, E. and KOFOID, C.A. (1938). THE RELATIONSHIP OF HEXAMITA SP. TO AN ENTERITIS OF TURKEY POULTS. Cornell Vet. 28: 281-293.

(22) ITAGAKI, SHIRO (1927). ON THE LIFE HISTORY OF THE CHICKEN NEMATODE, ASCARIDIA PERSPICILLUM. 3d World's Poultry Cong. Proc., pp. 339-344, illus.

(23) JOHNSON, E.P. (1939). A METHOD OF RAISING TURKEYS IN CONFINEMENT TO PREVENT PARASITIC DISEASES. Va. Agr. Expt. Sta. Bull. 323, 16 pp.

(24) _____UNDERHILL, G.W., Cox, J.A. and THRELKELD, W.L. (1938). A BLOOD PROTOZOON OF TURKEYS TRANSMITTED BY SIMUDIUM NIGROPARVUM (TWINN). Amer. Jour. Hyg. 27: 649-665, illus.

(25) JONES, MYRNA F. (1936). METROLIASTHES LUCIDA, A CESTODE OF GALLIFORM BIRDS, IN ARTHROPOD AND AVIAN HOSTS. Helminthol. Soc. Wash. Proc. 3: 26-30, illus.

(26) _____and HORSFALL, M.W. (1935). ANTS AS INTERMEDIATE HOSTS FOR TWO SPECIES OF RAILLIETINA PARASITIC IN CHICKENS. Jour. Parasitol. 27: 442-443.

(27) _____and HORSFALL, MARGERY W. (1936). THE LIFE HISTORY OF A POULTRY CESTODE. Science 83; 303-804.

(28) JOYEUX, CHARLES and BAER, JEAN GEORGES (1937). BECHERCHES SUR L'EVOLUTION DES CESTODES DE GALLINACES. [Paris] Acad. des Sci. Compt. Rend. 205: 751-753.

(29) JUNGHERR, ERWIN (1927). TWO INTERESTING TURKEY DISEASES. Amer. Vet. Med. Assoc. Jour. 71; 636-640, illus.

(30) KOTLAN, A. and CHANDLER, W..L. (1925). A NEWLY RECOGNIZED FLUKE DISEASE (PROSTHOGONIMIASIS) OF FOWLS IN THE UNITED STATES. Amer. Vet. Med. Assoc. Jour. 67: 756- 763, illus.

(31) _____and CHANDLER, W.L. (1927). ON THE ROLE PLAYED BY DRAGONFLIES IN THE TRANSFER OF PROSTHOGONIMUS. Amer. Vet. Med. Assoc. Jour. 70: 520-524.

(32) LEVINE, NORMAN D., BOLEY, L.E. and HESTER, H.R. (1941). EXPERIMENTAL TRANSMISSION OF TRICHOMONAS GALLINAE FROM THE CHICKEN TO OTHER BIRDS. Amer. Jour. Hyg., Sect. C. 33: 23-32.

(33) _____and BRANDLY, C.A. (1939). A PATHOGENIC TRICHOMONAS FROM THE UPPER DIGESTIVE TRACT OF CHICKENS. Amer. Vet. Med. Assoc. Jour. 95. 77-78, illus.

(34) LEVINE, P.P. (1938). INFECTION OF THE CHICKEN WITH CAPILLARIA COLUMBAE (Rud.). Jour. Parasitol. 24; [45]-52.

(35) MACY, RALPH W. (1934). PROSTHOGONIMUS MACRORCHIS N. SP., THE COMMON OVIDUCT FLUKE OF DOMESTIC FOWLS IN THE NORTHERN UNITED STATES. Amer. Micros. Soc. Trans. 53; 30—34, illus.

(36) _____(1934). STUDIES ON THE TAXONOMY, MORPHOLOGY AND BIOLOGY OF PROSTHOGONIMUS MACRORCHIS MACY, A COMMON OVIDUCT FLUKE OF DOMESTIC FOWLS IN NORTH AMERICA. Minn. Agr. Expt. Sta. Tech. Bull. 98, 71 pp., illus.

(37) McCULLOCH, ERNEST C. and NICHOLSON, LYLE G. (1940). PHENOTHIAZINE FOR THE REMOVAL OF HETERAKIS GALLINAE FROM CHICKENS. Vet. Med. 35: 398-400, illus.

(38) OLSEN, MARLOW W. and ALLEN, ENA A. (1940). TREATMENT OF CECAL AND LIVER TRICHOMONIASIS IN TURKEYS BY FEVER THERAPY. (Preliminary paper) Soc. Expt. Biol. and Med. Proc. 45; 875-876.

(39) O'ROKE, EARL C. (1934). A MALARIA-LIKE DISEASE OF DUCKS CAUSED BY LEUCOOYTOZOON ANATIS WICKWARE. Mich. Univ. School Forestry and Conserv. Bull. 4, 44 pp., illus.

(40) ROBERTS, F.H.S. (1940). A PRELIMINARY NOTE ON THE EFFICIENCY OF PHENOTHIAZINE AGAINST SOME POULTRY HELMINTHS. Austral. Vet. Jour. 16: 172-174.

(41) SANDERS, D.A. (1928). MANSON'S EYEWORM OF POULTRY. Amer. Vet. Med. Assoc. Jour. 72; 568-584, illus.

(42) SKIDMORE, LOIUS V. (1932). LEUCOCYTOZOON SMITHI INFECTION IN TURKEYS AND ITS TRANSMISSION BY SIMULIUM OCCIDENTALE TOWNSEND. Zentbl. f. Bakt. [etc.] Originale (I) 125: 829-335, illus.

(43) STABLER, ROBERT M. (1938). THE SIMILARITY BETWEEN THE FLAGELLATE OF TURKEY TRICHOMONIASIS AND T. COLUMBAE IN THE PIGEON. Amer. Vet. Med. Assoc. Jour. 93: 33-34, illus.

(44) _____(1938). TRICHOMONAS GALLINAE BIVOLTA, (1878) THE CORRECT NAME FOR THE FLAGELLATE IN THE MOUTH, CROP AND LIVER OF THE PIGEON. (Research note) Jour. Parasitol. 24: 558-554.

(45) TYZZER, ERNEST EDWARD (1927). ENTERO-HEPATITIS IN TURKEYS AND ITS TRANSMISSION THROUGH THE AGENCY OF HETERAKIS VESICULASIS. 3d World's Poultry Cong. 1- Proc., pp. 286-200, illus.

(46) _____(1934). STUDIES ON HISTOMONIASIS, OR "BLACKHEAD" INFECTION, IN THE CHICKEN AND TURKEY. Amer. Acad. Arts and Sci. Proc. 69: [189]-264, illus.

(47) _____and FABYAN, M. (1920). FURTHER STUDIES ON "BLACKHEAD" IN TURKEYS, WITH SPECIAL REFERENCE TO TRANSMISSION BY INOCULATION. Jour. Infect. Dis. 27; [207]-289, illus.

(48) UDERHILL, G.W. (1939). TWO SIMULIDS FOUND FEEDING ON TURKEYS IN VIRGINIA. Ent. 32: 765-768.

(49) VOLKMAR, FRITZ (1930). TRICHOMONAS DIVERSA N. SP. AND ITS ASSOCIATION WITH A DISEASE OF TURKEYS. Jour. Parasitol. 17: [85]-89, illus.

(50) WEHR, EVERETT E. (1936). EARTHWORMS AS TRANSMITTERS OF CAPILLARIA ANNULATA, THE "CROP-WORM" OF CHICKENS. North Amer. Vet. 17 (8): 18-20, illus.

(51) _____(1937). RELATIVE ABUNDANCE OF CROP WORMS IN TURKEYS: MACROSCOPIC DIFFERENTIATION OF SPECIES. Vet: Med. 32: 230-233, illus.

(52) _____(1939). THE GAPEWORM AS A MENACE TO POULTRY PRODUCTION. 7th World's Poultry Cong. Proc., pp. 267-270.

(52a)_____(1939). STUDIES ON THE DEVELOPMENT OF THE PIGEON CAPILLARID, CAPILLARIA COLUMBAE. U.S. Dept. Agr. Tech. Bull. 679, 19 pp., illus.

(53) ____HARWOOD, PAUL D. and SCHAFFER, JACOB M. (1939). BARIUM ANTIMONYI, TARTRATE AS A REMEDY FOR THE REMOVAL OF GAPEWORMS FROM CHICKENS. Poultry Sci. 18; 63-65.

Chapter 8

COCCIDIOSIS OF THE CHICKEN

John F. Christensen & Ena A. Allen[1]

[1] *John F. Christensen and Ena A. Allen are Associate Protozoologists Zoological Division, Bureau of Animal Industry.*

Ann account of the life history, symptoms of infection and methods of control of a group of internal parasites that are among the most serious enemies of poultry production.

"It is probable that coccidia cause greater economic loss among domesticated animals of the temperate zone than any other group of protozoa." Thus Becker[2] aptly indicated the importance of coccidiosis, the specific disease caused by these protozoan parasites. It may be added that the coccidia probably cause greater economic loss; among chickens alone than among all other domesticated animals combined, despite the fact that coccidiosis occurs frequently in severe outbreaks among other domesticated fowl, cattle and sheep and occasionally among goats, pigs and dogs. Because of the preponderant significance of the disease in chickens, this article is confined to a description of the coccidia and coccidiosis of these birds. However, the life histories of the parasites, the nature of the disease and the principles of control are essentially similar for all domesticated and semi-domesticated fowl and the information given therefore applies in general also to coccidiosis of the duck, goose,

[2] BECKER, ELERY R. COCCIDIA AND COCCIDIOSIS OF DOMESTICATED, GAME AND LABORATORY ANIMALS AND OF MAN. 147 pp., Illus. Awes, Iowa. 1934.

guinea fowl, pheasant, pigeon, quail and turkey, all of which harbour, characteristic kinds or species of coccidia.

The Life History of a Poultry Coccidium

The coccidia belong to a group of Protozoa known as Sporozoa, so designated because they produce sporelike infective bodies at some stage in their life histories. Resistant cysts–enclosed, egglike forms–of these parasites are discharged from their hosts in the feces or droppings and must pass through a process of development called sporulation in the outside environment before being infective to other animals. With the exception of *Tyzzeria* of the duck, the coccidia of the chicken and all other barnyard fowls belong to the genus *Eimeria*, the life histories of all species of which are in general similar.

The life history may be said to begin with the discharge of the microscopic, egglike, resistant forms known as oöcysts in the droppings of infected birds. Under conditions of optimum moisture, moderate temperature and ample oxygen supply, these eliminated oöcysts sporulate within a few days. This process consists in division of the protoplasm within each oöcyst shell into four elongated bodies, each in turn secreting its own shell, within which the protoplasm again divides to form two comma-shaped or sausage-shaped sporozoites. Each sporulated oöcyst thus contains eight sporozoites, which are infective agents capable of giving rise to coccidial infection when swallowed by susceptible birds.

Sporulated oöcysts may be ingested by susceptible birds soon after development is complete, or they may lie dormant for months in litter or soil, if temperature and moisture are favorable, before being picked up by new hosts. Once eaten by a susceptible bird, the oöcysts are in some way activated the intestine of the host so that the sporozoites are released into the intestinal canal. The liberated sporozoites are capable of slow flexing movements and when they come in contact with the intestinal wall in certain regions of the alimentary tract they penetrate cell membranes and enter the living protoplasm.

Inside the host cells the sporozoites lose their ability to move around and they grow at the expense of the parasitized cells. After a definite period of growth the protoplasm of each parasite divides into many small, elongated bodies known as merozoites, which are expelled from the tissue by rupture of the cell membranes. These merozoites also possess limited powers of locomotion and immediately parasitize other cells. Again there is growth and multiplication, with the production of additional swarms of merozoites. After two or more generations of such a sexual reproduction, some of the merozoites become sexually differentiated after entering new cells. The female parasites are large, rounded and inactive. The male parasite produces by segmentation vast numbers of extremely small, actively moving bodies each capable of activating or fertilizing a single female parasite. After fertilization and secretion of a resistant shell, the female parasites are extruded, or pushed out, from the damaged host tissue into the alimentary stream and discharged from the host birds in the droppings, being then designated as oöcysts.

Cecal Coccidiosis

There are two distinct types of coccidiosis of the chicken, depending upon the site of localization and multiplication of the parasites in the digestive tracts of the infected birds. In cecal coccidiosis, the coccidia invade the mucous membrane of the ceca, or blind guts, of chicks (Fig. 1), producing as a result of rapid multiplication and extensive destruction of tissue an acute and often highly fatal disease characterized by severe cecal hemorrhage. In the intestinal disease, the parasites become localized largely in the small intestine and give rise to a serious but usually less acute infection of older, maturing birds sometimes characterized by extreme wasting flesh and slow, insidious development.

Cecal coccidiosis is primarily a disease of, chicks 3 to 5 weeks old, although infection may occur in birds of any age. The disease usually strikes rather suddenly producing illness or death in a considerable number of chicks at about the same time. In severe infections, many birds may die suddenly without showing visible symptoms, but they usually have pale combs and some blood on the feathers surrounding the vent and when the birds are opened for examination, the ceca are found to be bulging with blood. Other birds have a ruffled, droopy appearance (Fig. 2), lose appetite, fall off rapidly in weight, have a subnormal temperature, show pale skin and mucous membranes as a result of cecal hemmorrhage and discharge bloody droppings. Some of these sick birds die during the first few days of illness, while others linger for several days to a week or more before finally succumbing to emaciation or wasting of

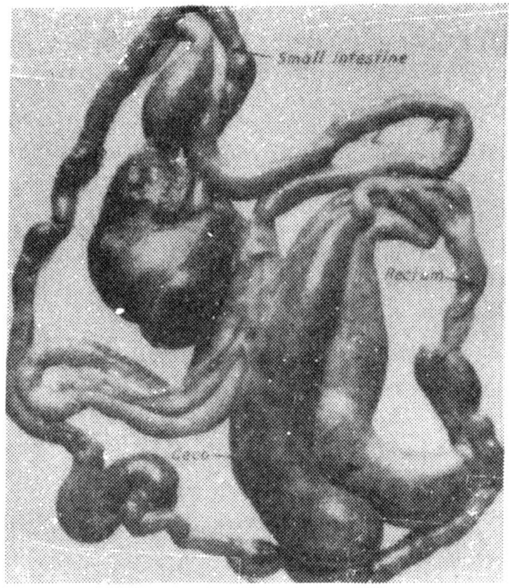

Fig. 1: Viscera of a chicken that died from an infection of *Eimeria tenella*. Note ceca distended with blood.

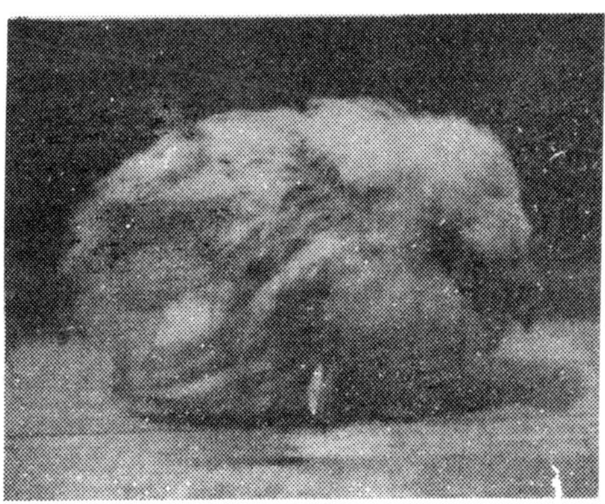

Fig. 2: Chicken suffering from an attack of cecal coccidiosis.

flesh and loss of blood. With good care, many sick chicks gradually overcome the pallor, regain flesh and recover.

Tyzzer[3] demonstrated that cecal coccidiosis is caused by a single species of coccidium, *Eimeria tenella*. The information he obtained from study with experimentally infected birds provided the basis for a complete understanding of the natural disease. On the fourth day after inoculation with heavy doses of sporulated oöcysts of *E. tenella*, birds show symptoms of severe cecal coccidiosis and when they are killed for examination, bleeding from the cecal walls has begun. The greatest number of deaths occur on the fifth and sixth days of infection, when cecal hemorrhage reaches its peak, the birds show pale skin and mucous membranes from loss of blood and the droppings contain blood. Chicks that die during the period of greatest hemorrhage have ceca bulging with fluid blood (Fig. 1). When death occurs later in the infection, the blood and tissue debris in the ceca have formed clotted or cheesy cores, while the cecal walls appear thickened and mottled from hemorrhage and the tissues and organs are pale from loss of blood. It was demonstrated that the widespread leakage of blood from the cecal mucous membrane during the infection results from the destruction of tissue by the maturing second generation parasites and the liberation of enormous numbers of second generation merozoites.

Intestinal Coccidiosis

Although usually less acute and spectacular in its onset than the cecal infection, intestinal coccidiosis causes a tremendous economic loss to poultry farmers by making heavy inroads on flocks of maturing chickens at a time when considerable cash outlay is represented. Of the six well-established species of coccidia that become localized in the small intestine of chickens, *Eimeria nectrix* is the one responsible for severe clinical intestinal coccidiosis, although other species have been demonstrated by experimental infections to produce less severe clinical symptoms. Thus, *E. acervulina* may produce coccidiosis of long duration characterized by extreme emaciation and *E. maxima* causes thickening of the intestinal wall and produces a slight hemorrhage from the damaged mucous membrane in very heavy infections.

---

[3] TYZZER, ERNEST EDWARD. COCCIDIOSIS IN GALLINACEOUS BIRDS. Amer. Jour. Hyg. 10: 269-383, illus. 1929.

This type of coccidiosis is primarily a disease of maturing birds and frequently appears soon after pullets are confined to laying houses. The infection is first recognized in only a few birds of a flock, but additional individuals develop symptoms from day to day until considerable numbers are affected. The symptoms are in general similar to those noted for chicks with cecal coccidiosis, consisting in droopiness, a ruffled appearance, loss of appetite, increasing emaciation and weakness and pallor resulting from intestinal hemorrhage. Death from the disease may occur during the early stages of the attack, but usually only after several days to 2 or 3 weeks of illness. Many sick birds gradually regain their appetite and strength and recover from the attack.

As Tyzzer had done previously for *Eimeria tenella*, Tyzzeri Theiler and Jones[4] worked out the intricate details of the life history of *E. necatrix* and the course of experimental infection in the chicken in order to obtain the information essential for an accurate conception of the natural disease. They demonstrated that susceptible chickens experimentally infected with large single dosages of sporulated oöcysts of *E. necatrix* show the first symptoms of coccidiosis at the end of 4 days of infection. The heaviest death losses occur on the sixth and seventh days of infection as a result of the destruction of tissue and the bleeding produced by the action of the parasites in the intestinal mucous membrane. The unopened small intestine of birds that die at the height of infection appears heavily peppered with small opaque spots and hemorrhagic blotched and streaks, especially in the middle portion (Fig. 3). Microscopic study reveals that these opaque spots or lesions are large colonies of maturing second-generation parasites located deep in the mucous membrane and that the bleeding commences at the centres of these lesions in the tissue destroyed by the parasites. The affected intestine is congested with blood and is flabby, distended and easily ruptured; it is filled with material varying from a clear, jellylike, yellowish exudate to clotted blood, which often forms a solid, fibrinous cylinder completely blocking the intestinal canal. During the sixth day, the muscular function of the intestine is usually completely lost as a

[4] TYZZER, ERNEST E., THEILER, HANS, and JONES, E. ELIZABETH. COCCIDIOSIS IN GALLINACEOUS BIRDS. II. A COMPARATIVE STUDY OF SPECIES OF EIMERIA OF THE CHICKEN. J Amer. Jour. Hyg. 15: 319-393, illus. 1932.

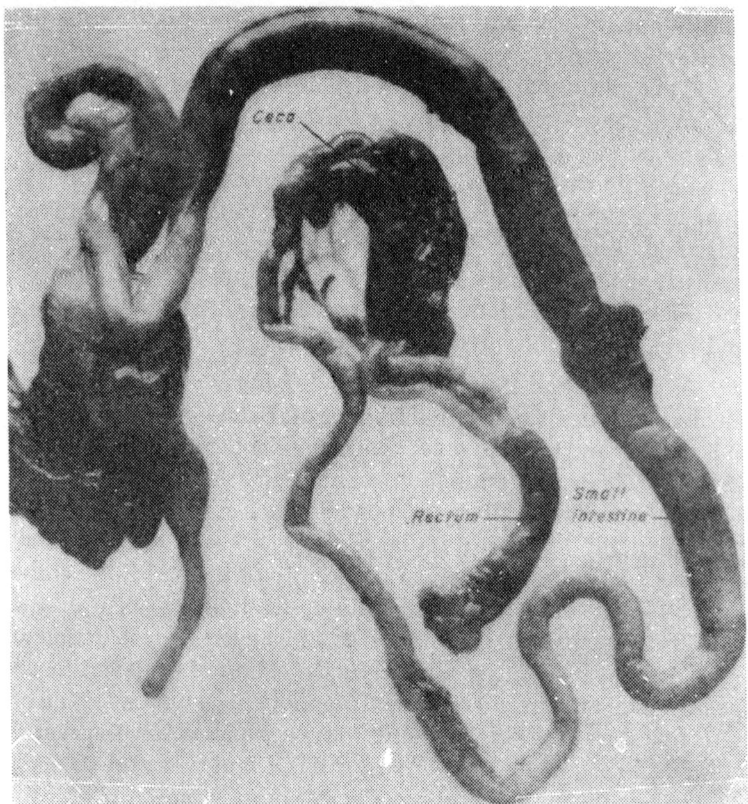

Fig. 3: Viscera of a chicken that died from an infection of *Eimeria necatrix*. Note that the entire small intestine as well as the ceca is affected.

result of obstruction with these massess of clotted tissue, exudate and blood. Birds that survive the seventh day of these heavy experimental infections usually recover. Within a day or two the intestine resumes functioning and the recovering chickens begin discharging watery droppings containing blood, mucus and occasional cylindrical masses of clotted material. Gradually the droppings become normal, appetite returns and paleness disappears, but the birds may remain extremely emaciated from malnutrition.

Control of Coccidiosis of the Chicken

Unfortunately, losses from coccidiosis do not cease with the deaths and sickness that result from an outbreak. According to Tyzzer, the damage resulting from severe infections to the ceca and intestine sometimes results in the permanent loss of function of considerable areas of mucous membrane in recovered chickens and this contributes to the chronic unthriftiness of many of these birds. Such fowls not only mature more slowly but produce fewer eggs during maturity than similar chickens that have had no early attack of clinical coccidiosis.[5] These are effects of the disease emphasize the wisdom of prevention as a means of control.

It is well established[6] that if reinfection is prevented, the coccidial parasites run fairly rapid, definite courses of multiplication within the host birds and are soon eliminated as oöcysts; that birds surviving severe or continued mild infections are subsequently resistant or immune to severe reinfections with the same species of coccidia; and that such immune adult birds are healthy carriers of coccidia and thus possible sources of infection of young stock. Prevention is based on these facts, which at once suggest that the supply of infective oöcysts should be kept as low as possible by application of rigid sanitation and that young susceptible birds should be kept strictly isolated from adult fowls.

Floors, walls, windows and equipment of brooder houses should be cleaned thoroughly with soap and hot water before the birds are admitted. After that the floors should be thoroughly dry-cleaned with a scuffle hoe and a stiff broom at least twice weekly until the birds are 10 or 12 weeks old, then weekly until they are transferred to laying houses. Dry cleaning prevents the accumulation of moisture, which favors the sporulation of oöcysts. Fresh, clean litter should be put in after each cleaning. If chicks are kept in cages, cleaning should be done daily, if possible. Feeding and watering equipment should be cleaned frequently and should be designed to prevent accumulations of moisture on floors or contamination of feed and drinking water with infective material.

---

[5] MAYHEW, ROY L. STUDIES ON COCCIDIOSIS. VI. EFFECTS OF EARLY ATTACK ON EGG PRODUCTION. Poultry Sci. 13: 148-154, illus. 1934.

[6] JOHNSON, W.T. COCCIDIOSIS OF THE CHICKEN. Oreg. AGr. Expt. Sta. Bul. 238, 16 pp., illus. 1928. See also the citation in footnote 3.

If there is enough land available, it is wise to use movable brooder houses that can be transferred occasionally to new ground stationary brooder houses should be located on well-drained, preferably sandy soil, which provides the quick-drying terrain least favorable for oöcyst development. It has been recommended that stationary brooder houses be provided with. sloping concrete runs, which can be covered lightly with sand and cleaned thoroughly at the same time; the houses are cleaned. During the period of confinement to laying houses special care must be taken to prevent conditions that would favour the development of intestinal coccidiosis among the pullets. The laying houses should be cleaned thoroughly before occupancy and frequently thereafter, in order that accumulations of moisture and litter, which favour oöcyst development, may be avoided. The same attention to sanitation should be given to the feeding and watering equipment for these older birds as to those for the brooding stock. If considerable range is available, clean ground should be provided for each group of pullets. At all times, the feeding, watering and cleaning equipment for young and adult stock should be kept separated in order to prevent any significant transfer of infective material to susceptible birds. Though strict application of these sanitary measures in the handling of young birds cannot be expected to eliminate coccidial infection completely, it should permit successful rearing.

Even when excellent care is provided, outbreaks of coccidiosis occur occasionally among young birds and at these times there is a demand for an immediate remedy. It is the general opinion among qualified authorities on poultry coccidiosis that there is little value in medicinal treatment of sick birds during an outbreak and that effort is applied more profitably in proper management. Early diagnosis and prompt adjustments in the feeding and care of birds are important. It is wise to segregate sick chickens provide warm quarters, avoid overcrowding, supply appetizing, easily digested, nutritious feed and redouble efforts at sanitation in order to remove oöcysts, which are shed in the droppings of sick birds in enormous numbers. Meticulous attention to all details of good feeding and care of sick birds may be expected to minimize losses during an outbreak, but treatment "can be recommended only as a means of making the best of an already bad situation, not as a routine preventive"[7].

---

[7] See reference in footnote 6.

Chapter 9

POULTRY LICE AND THEIR CONTROL

F.C. Bishopp[1]

[1] *F.C. Bishopp is Assistant Chief of the Bureau of Entomology and Plant Quarantine.*

Several different kinds of biting and chewing lice infest poultry, each having its preferred location on certain parts of the body. Young birds especially can be seriously affected or even killed by severe attacks. The delousing procedure described in this article can easily be applied on any farm.

Poultrymen realize that it is essential to control poultry lice, particularly in the case of chickens. These parasites are also a problem to those who raise turkeys, ducks, geese, guineas and pigeons or grow wild birds, such as quail and grouse, in captivity. Losses due to poultry lice throughout the United States run high in the millions of dollars each year as the result of death, especially among young fowls, retarded development, reduced egg production, interference with incubation and damage to plumage. Probably the losses are heaviest among farm and backyard flocks kept as a side line rather than among commercial flocks, which are given special attention. Enough is known about lice and their control to make these losses totally unnecessary.

All lice infesting poultry and birds are of the biting and chewing, not the bloodsucking, kind. Some persons confuse lice with mites.

The latter suck blood, differ from lice in their habits and are controlled by different methods.

In general, each species of poultry lice is confined to a particular kind of poultry, but some pass readily from one kind of fowl to another, especially when the birds are closely associated. In this country, chickens are rather commonly infested with seven species of lice, turkeys with three, ducks and geese with three, pigeons with three and guinea fowl and peafowl with two or three each.

Development and Habits of Poultry Lice

All species of poultry lice have certain habits in common. All of them live continuously on feathered hosts and soon die if removed from them. The eggs are attached to the feathers and the young lice closely resemble the adults except in colour and size. All poultry lice have strong chewing jaws, flattened bodies, legs fitted for clinging to feathers and a remarkable ability to move about and hide among the feathers.

They differ, however, in their preferred locations on the body and the feathers and these preferences have given rise to the common names applied to the various species.

The length of the incubation and development periods of several of the species have not been determined, but they are believed not to vary widely. In general it may be said that the incubation period ranges from 4 to 7 days. and the development of the lice from hatching to the adult stage requires 17 to 21 days. As the lice grow, the skins are shed two or three times. Mating takes place on the fowl and egg laying begins 2 or 3 days after the lice mature. The number of eggs deposited has not been accurately determined but appears to range from 50 to 300.

Chicken Lice

The Head Louse

As the name "head louse" suggests, this species (*Lipeurus heterographus*) is found mainly on the head, although it occurs occasionally on the neck and elsewhere. It is usually located close to the skin in the down or at the base of the feathers on the top and back of the head and beneath the bill. In fact, the head of the louse is often found so close to the skin that poultrymen think it is actually attached to the skin or is sucking blood. Although it does not suck blood, it is very irritating and ranks first among the lice as a pest of young chickens and turkeys, which often become infested within a few hours after hatching by lice from the mother. In cases of heavy infestation the chicks soon become droopy and weak and may die before they are a month old. When the chickens become fairly well feathered, head lice decrease in numbers, but they may increase again when the fowls reach maturity.

This louse (Fig. 1) is oblong, grayish and about one-tenth of an inch in length. The pearly white eggs (Fig. 2) are attached singly to the down or at the base of the small feathers on the head. They hatch in 4 or 5 days into minute, pale, translucent lice, resembling the adults in shape.

The Body Louse

The body louse (*Menacanthus stramineus*) of chickens prefers to stay on the skin rather than on the feathers and it chooses parts of the body that are not densely feathered, such as the area below the vent. In heavy infestations it may be found on the breast, under the wings and on other parts of the body, including even the head.

When the feathers are parted, the straw-coloured body lice may be seen running rapidly on the skin in search of cover. The eggs are deposited in clusters near the base of small feathers, particularly below the vent or, in young fowls, frequently on the head or along the throat. The eggs hatch in about a week and the lice reach maturity in 17 to 20 days.

This is the most important of the lice that infest grown chickens. When it is present in large numbers, the skin is greatly irritated and scabs may result, especially below the vent.

The Shaft Louse

The shaft louse, or small body louse (*Menopon gallinae*), is similar in appearance to the body louse but somewhat smaller. It has a habit of resting on the shafts of the body feathers of chickens, where it may be seen running rapidly toward the body when the feathers are suddenly parted. Sometimes as many as a dozen lice may be seen scurrying downward along a feather shaft.

Since the shaft louse apparently feeds only on parts of the feathers, it is much less important than its relative, the body louse. It is found in limited numbers on turkeys, guinea fowl and ducks kept

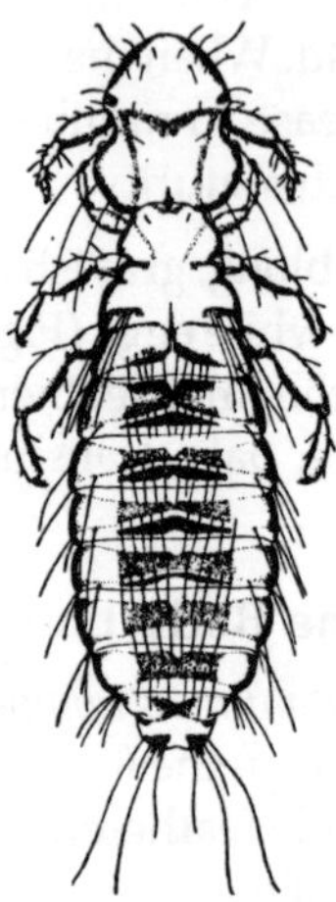

Fig. 1: Head louse of the chicken, adult male. Greatly enlarged.

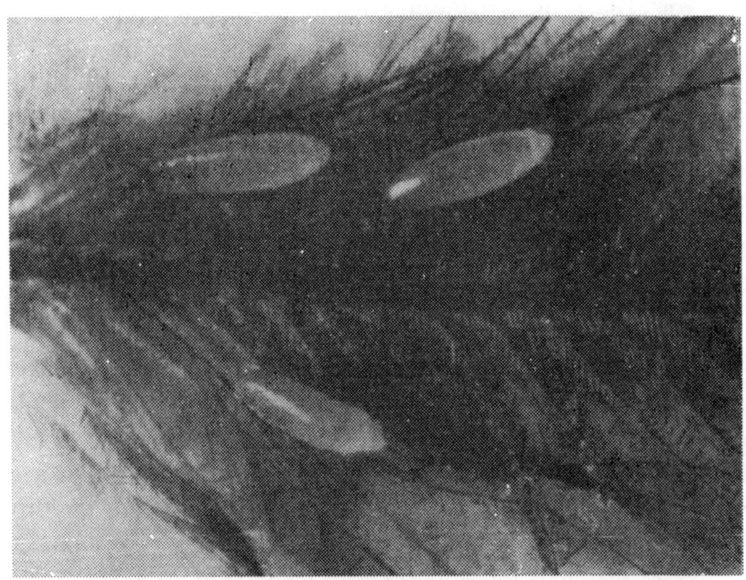

Fig. 2: Eggs of the head louse of the chicken. Greatly enlarged.

in close association with chickens. It does not stay on young birds until they become well feathered.

Other Kinds of Chicken Lice

Four other kinds of lice are found rather commonly on chickens, but they are usually less abundant and important than those just discussed. The wing louse (*Lipeurus caponis*), a slender gray species resembling the head louse, to which it is related, is the most widely distributed and is found in the greatest numbers. It is sluggish and is usually seen resting between the barbules of the wing and tail feathers, or occasionally on the neck hackles and feathers of the back.

The fluff louse (*Goniocotes hologaster*), which is found, as the common Dame implies, on the fluff of the body feathers, is small, rather broad, yellow in colour and inactive. As it stays mostly in the fluff, it causes little irritation or other injury.

The large chicken louse (*Goniocotes gigas*) is a robust, dark, smoky-gray species of striking appearance. It is seldom abundant or of much importance.

The brown chicken louse (*Goniodes dissimilis*), occurring mainly in the Southern States, is large and reddish brown in colour. It seldom occurs in large enough numbers to cause serious damage.

Turkey Lice

The slender turkey louse (*Lipeurus gallipavonis*) and the large turkey louse (*Goniodes meleagridis*) are found on both wild and domesticated turkeys and may cause serious annoyance, although as a rule they are not very abundant. Poults hatched by chickens are often infested with the common body louse and the head louse, which pass to them from the foster mother. The combined attacks of these lice may retard growth and reduce the vigor of young turkeys. Head lice have been reported to have caused heavy mortality among newly hatched poults.

Lice of Geese, Ducks, Pigeons and Poultry

Geese and ducks are seldom noticeably affected by lice. Three of four species are occasionally found on these fowls and when the young are hatched by hens they are often attacked by the head louse of chickens.

Pigeons are subject to the attacks of six species of lice. Some of these are to be found on the birds in practically every pigeon loft, but they seldom become sufficiently abundant to cause marked in effects. Carrier pigeons and show birds frequently have damaged feathers and some owners attribute this to lice, particularly the large body louse (Fig. 3). The damage in such cases adversely affects the appearance of the birds and probably also their speed and endurance in flight.

Control Measures

Since all bird lice live continuously and breed on the plumage and bodies of their hosts, little attention need be paid in control operations to the houses, litter and yards. In eradicating lice all poultry on the premises should be regarded as lousy if any of them have lice.

In general it is advisable to delouse a flock in the fall when the surplus stock is disposed of so that the number of fowls to be treated is reduced. This assures their entering the winter free from lice. If no infested fowls are added to the flock, it will be free from the pests the following spring, which is especially desirable where hens are used for hatching and brooding.

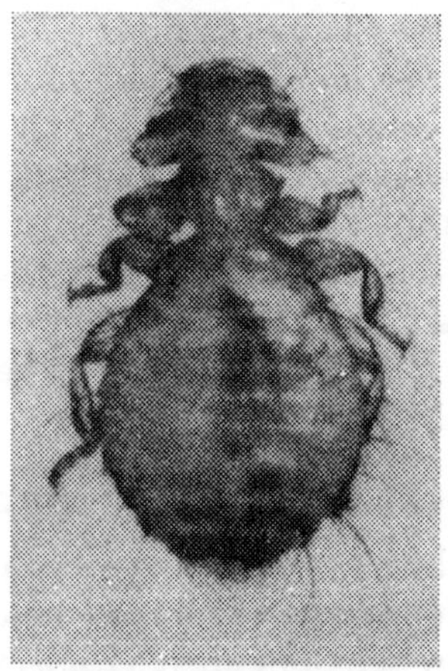

Fig. 3: The large body louse of pigeons. Enlarged.

Fortunately control procedures have been developed that are highly effective and thoroughly practical.

Sodium Fluoride Versus Lice

Methods of eradicating poultry lice through the use of sodium fluoride as a powder or a dip were first described in 1917.[2] A single treatment will destroy all species of lice, including all eggs, without injury to the fowls.

Commercial sodium fluoride is recommended for this purpose. It is a white powder which should contain 90 to 98 percent sodium fluoride. The material is generally available and usually retails at 30 to 60 cents a pound. *Since sodium fluoride is poisonous to human beings and animals when taken internally, care should be exercised in storing the powder, so that it will not be mistaken for something else and in disposing of solutions of it.*

To insure treatment of all louse carriers the fowls should be shut up at night and a search made for any that do not roost in the poultry house.

Dusting

The lice are found on various parts of the body and it is essential that the sodium fluoride be placed on the infested areas. With this method it is necessary for two people to work together, one holding the fowl and the other applying the insecticide. The powder may be applied with a shaker can held in one hand while with the other the feathers are raised so the powder will reach the skin. It is best to hold the birds over a shallow pan to catch the surplus powder. It is also economical to dilute the powder by adding 2 parts of some fine material, such as flour, road dust, or sulfur, to 1 part of sodium fluoride.

The so-called pinch method is preferable to the use of a shaker. It involves less waste and less dust floating in the air and only one operator is required. The fowl is held in one hand by grasping the base of the wings over the back and the powder, kept in a pan near at hand, is applied by placing a small pinch among the feathers next to the skin. About 11 pinches are applied to the fowl, 2 along

---

2 BISHOPP, F.C., and WOOD, H.P. MITES AND LICE ON POULTRY. U.S. Dept. Agr. Farmers' Bul. 801, 27 pp., illus. 1917. (Revised, 1939).

the back, 1 on the neck, 1 on the head, 1 on the breast, 1 below the vent, 1 on each thigh, 1 on the tail and 1 on each wing when spread.

Since sodium fluoride is irritating to the nose and throat, the operator should wear a respirator or a piece of wet cloth over his nose and mouth. The fowls should be released in the open air as fast as they are treated.

Young chickens and other fowls are likely to be injured if they are hovered closely by the mother after she has been treated. It is therefore highly advisable to delouse hens before the young hatch. If this has not been done, the young should not be treated until they are a week old and then only two very small pinches of the powder should be applied to each, one distributed on the back, neck and head and the other on the under side, including the throat.

Grown turkeys should receive about 15 pinches of the powder and pigeons 5. Because of the close feathers of the latter, however, dipping is more effective.

Dipping

Some poultry raisers maintain that fowls should not be dipped. Extensive experience, however, has shown that when more than 35 fowls are to be treated, dipping in sodium fluoride solution is highly effective, economical, convenient and without ill effects on the poultry. The only precautions necessary are that the birds should be handled carefully, that the work should be done on a mild sunny day or in a warm poultry house and that the operation should be completed at least an hour before sundown. Fowls dipped in the solution are not thoroughly wet and the feathers dry in an hour or two.

The procedure is simple. Tepid water is measured into a tub and a rounded tablespoonful of sodium fluoride is added for each gallon. The solution should be within 6 or 8 inches of the top of the tub, which is then placed on a box at a convenient height for dipping. The fowls are held in one hand by the wings over the back and lowered into the solution, with the head left out above it. The feathers are, then raised beneath the solution with the other hand to allow penetration, the head is ducked and the fowl is lifted out, allowed to drain a few seconds and liberated. The actual dipping of a fowl requires only 20 to 30 seconds.

To completely rid pigeons of lice it is necessary to add 1 ounce of laundry soap to the dip to obtain a complete wetting of the feathers.[3]

Cost of Treatment

One pound of sodium fluoride applied by the pinch method will treat about 100 hens. When a considerable number of fowls are to be treated, less than half that amount is required for dipping. Figuring the powder at 40 cents a pound and the labour at 30 cents an hour, the cost for treating 100 fowls amounts to $1.65 by the pinch method and $1 by the dipping method. This is very reasonable when it is considered that one treatment means the complete eradication of all lice from the premises, provided all the fowls are treated.

Other Remedies

Nicotine sulfate applied to the roosts under proper conditions is reasonably effective in eradicating lice. The pure (40 percent) material is applied with a brush to the upper side of the roosts about half an hour before the fowls go to roost. The fumes penetrate the feathers and the lice continue to die and drop out during several nights following the application. This method works best in reasonably tight chicken houses and during warm weather. It cannot be depended on to eradicate lice completely, however, as it does not reach all of them, especially those on the head and usually some of the fowls do not roost on the treated perches.

Sodium fluosilicate, a compound related to sodium fluoride, is a satisfactory substitute when used as a dip in the same way as the latter. The material is usually too coarse for very effective use as a dust.

Fine sulfur applied freely as a dust has been found satisfactory as a control for poultry lice. In order to destroy all the parasites in a single treatment, the treatment must be very thorough.

Many other materials and mixtures will destroy poultry lice, but everything considered, none is equal to sodium fluoride. Dust

---

[3] WOOD, H.P. THE ERADICATION OF LICE ON PIGEONS. U.S. Dept. Agr. Dept. Cir. 213, 4 pp. 1992.

baths are useful in holding down louse infestations, but some fowls do not use such baths and elimination of lice is never accomplished by this means.

Some remedies offered for sale and even widely used have little or no value in louse control. Among these should be mentioned materials sold for putting in the water or feed of poultry. Most of these are sulfur compounds. Such internal medication has been found to be valueless for the control of external parasites.

Chapter 10

POULTRY MITES

F.C. Bishopp[1]

[1] *F.C. Bishopp is Assistant Chief of the Bureau of Entomology and Plant Quarantine.*

Good poultry husbandry requires keeping the birds free of mites as far as possible, since these pests can do considerable damage. The remedies are simple and fairly easy to apply.

All classes of poultry are subject to the attack of mites, some of which are bloodsuckers, while others burrow in the skin or live on or in the feathers and still others occur in the air passage and in the lungs, liver and other internal organs.

The total loss chargeable to poultry mites is large, since these parasites cause retarded growth, reduced egg production, poor condition, lowered vitality, damaged plumage and even death. Much of the injury, consisting of constant irritation and loss of blood, is not apparent. A large percentage of the chickens, turkeys and other poultry throughout the country are more or less constantly infested with one or several kinds of mites. Some of the more important forms will be briefly discussed in this article and methods of combating them will be outlined.

The Chicken Mite

Most poultry raisers are familiar with the common chicken mite (*Dermanyssus gallinae*). This pest is present in all parts of the country and affects all kinds of poultry. It is a bloodsucker and, when present in large numbers, saps the vitality of the birds, the loss of blood and the irritation caused being sufficient to make the fowls anaemic, weak and restless. Egg production is seriously reduced, the eggs are spotted with mite excrement and setting hens are disturbed and may be driven off the nests so that the eggs do not hatch. Hens have been known to die from mite attacks while sitting on the nest and stock on feed fall to fatten. In addition, these mites may become annoying pests of human beings, especially persons who take care of poultry and livestock in buildings adjacent to poultry houses are also attacked.

The chicken mites are night raiders; for the most part they remain hidden away in cracks and crevices during the day. Hens on nests may be attacked during the day, however and on very heavily infested premises some mites are to be found among the feathers of the fowls during the day.

In all its active stages the mite sucks the blood of fowls, which is necessary to its development and reproduction. Usually the mites become engorged in a few minutes after inserting their beaks. They may bite the fowls on any part of the body. After feeding, the mites crawl off the host and seek a hiding place around the roosts or nests. When numerous, they may spread to the walls, floor and ceiling of the poultry house. About a day after feeding, the adult female mites deposit 3 to 7 pearly white eggs in the crack where they are hiding. As many as 8 clutches of eggs are deposited by each female, with a blood meal preceding each.

The eggs hatch in about 2 days and the young six-legged mite molts its skin without feeding and gains another pair of legs. The mite then feeds and molts its skin 1 or 2 days later this process is repeated once more and the mite is then mature. Since the cycle from egg to adult requires only about a week, multiplication can be very rapid under favorable conditions. During cold weather, development is slowed down and the life span is extended. An infested poultry house will remain infested 4 or 5 months after it is vacated and even longer in winter.

The chicken mite will feed freely on pigeons, canaries and wild birds such as sparrows. Wild birds are undoubtedly responsible for the spread of mites in some cases,. but such things as infested baskets and crates and even human carriers, are of much greater importance.

Since chicken mites hide during the daytime in cracks around the roosting and nesting places of the fowls, they may be eliminated by properly treating these places and without paying any attention to the fowls. The major difficulty is to reach the hidden mites. This requires thorough application of an effective and very penetrating insecticide.

The control methods recommended for the chicken mite are also effective against the fowl tick and the bedbug.

The first. step is to remove unnecessary boards, boxes and trash from the poultry house and yard. Next, remove and burn litter and nest material. Then apply one of the carbolineums (high-grade anthracene oil), crude petroleum, or creosote oil. If the house is very heavily infested, the entire interior, including the roof, should be sprayed. If the infestation is light, applying the material to the roosts, roost supports, nests,. and adjacent areas on the walls usually suffices.

General spray applications are best made with a bucket pump, knapsack sprayer, or barrel pump. A high pressure must be maintained and the spray material should be driven into all cracks. For light infestations a hand sprayer may be used, or the material may be applied with a brush.

The materials recommended have considerable penetrating power and persist well, so that if the application is thorough a single treatment will usually clear up the infestation. Occasionally a second application 3 or 4 weeks after the first is necessary and this may be made with a brush.

Since these materials stain and are somewhat caustic, care should be taken not to get them on the clothing, face, or body, or on the fowls. The spraying should be done early in the day so the material will have time to soak in before the fowls go to roost. It is advisable to clean out infestations before hens are set and to treat brooders and colony houses before they are used for young stock.

There are a number of other materials, such as kerosene-pyrethrum and nicotine sulfate, which if thoroughly and persistently used will clean up an infestation, but in the long run the materials first mentioned are usually more effective and cheaper. Whitewash is of some value in reducing mite infestations by sealing the mites in the cracks, but it will not accomplish complete control.

The Feather Mite

The feather mite (*Liponyssus sylviarum*) is an occasional but serious pest of chickens. Heavy infestations result in lowered condition of the birds and reduced egg production as well as a scabby condition of the skin and discolouration of the plumage. This mite remains on the fowls constantly and hence is more irritating to them than the common chicken mite.

Since the feather mite is found on a number of species of free-flying birds, including robins, swallows and sparrows, it seems almost certain that many of the infestations on poultry farms come from the contacts of these birds with the chickens.

The mite closely resembles the common chicken mite, but it is slightly smaller and somewhat more active. It can be differentiated from other mites by the fact that it is present in numbers on fowls in the daytime and causes a dirty appearance of the feathers (Fig. 1). It prefers the areas below the vent and around the tail, but in heavy infestations it occurs on the back and other parts and may also be seen running about on the eggs in the nests.

The female lays its eggs among the feathers, where the young mites hatch and complete their development without leaving the fowl.

Since the feather mite remains on the fowls most of the time, it is necessary to treat the fowls with an insecticide rather than to treat the roosts, as in the case of the chicken mite.

In view of the seriousness of the pest and the fact that it is not generally distributed among poultry, it should be completely eradicated before it spreads any further. In numerous instances eradication has been accomplished by the following procedure:

Dip every well-feathered fowl in a tub nearly filled with water to which 2 ounces of fine sulfur (98 percent passing a 325-mesh sieve) and 1 ounce of soap have been added for each gallon. Hold the fowl by the wings over the back and dip it, taking care to wet all the features thoroughly and duck the head also. Since this treatment makes all the feathers wet, it is necessary to do the work on a warm sunny day or in a heated building so that the birds will not be chilled while drying.

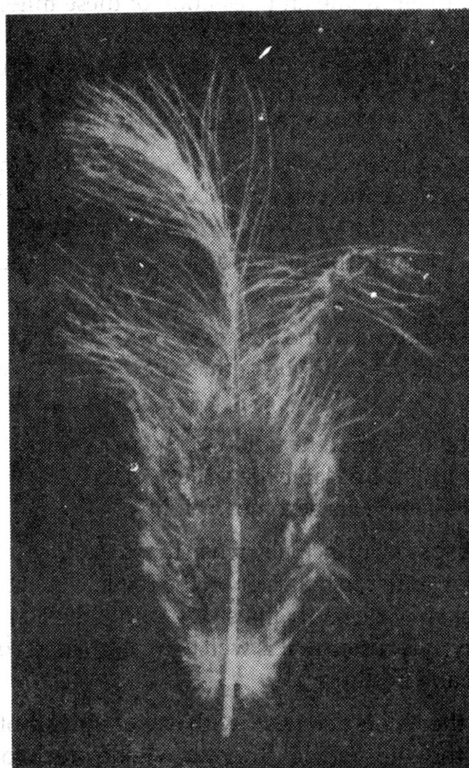

Fig. 1: Feather mites on a chicken feather.

If the outbreak occurs during the winter, complete destruction of all the mites on the fowls may be accomplished by dusting them thoroughly and freely with fine sulfur.

While the fowls are being treated, the nest material and litter should be removed and burned and the next boxes, walls and floors sprayed as recommended for control of the chicken mite.

Nests of English sparrows around the buildings should be pulled down and burned and these birds should be prevented from nesting about the premises.

Applying nicotine sulfate to the perches shortly before the fowls go to roost, as is sometimes done by controlling lice, has been found by Cleveland[2] to eliminate an infestation of these mites when it is done under favorable conditions. This treatment is especially useful during cold weather when dipping cannot be carried out.

The Scaly-Leg Mite

The scaly-leg mite (*Cnemidocoptes mutans*) commonly afflicts chickens throughout the country. In many instances, it does not cause serious injury, but when nothing is done to check it an attack may result in deformity of the feet and legs and even actual loss of the tips of the toes.

The parasite is one of the itch mites, living beneath and scales of the shanks and feet and also attaching the comb, wattles and neck.

At first the only manifestation of the trouble is the irritation shown by the fowls, but later the scales begin to thicken and rise and soon the feet and legs become unsightly.

The mites spread. principally when the fowls are in close contact with each other, either in crates or on the roost. Occasionally a few fowls in a flock may, be badly infested without the others showing material injury; nevertheless it is well to treat fowls as soon as there is evidence of an infestation.

Painting the roosts and nests with one of the carbolineums for the control of the common poultry mite will do much to reduce the spread of the scaly-leg mite. If only a few fowls show infestations they may be culled out and disposed of, or the legs may be dipped in crude petroleum (Fig. 2). Care should be taken not to permit the oil to get on the feathers and not to immerse the legs above the hock. One application is usually sufficient, but if most of the scales have not dropped off after a month, a second treatment should be given. Sometimes it is necessary to dip the legs of all the fowls in a flock. This should certainly be done if there is evidence of widespread infestation among them.

The Depluming Mite

Another mite, *Cnemidocoptes gallinae*, related to the scaly-leg mites frequently causes severe irritation by burrowing in the skin

---

[2] CLEVELAND, C.R. CONTROL OF POULTRY LICE AND MITES. Ind. Univ. Ext. Bul. 109, 8 pp. illus, 1922.

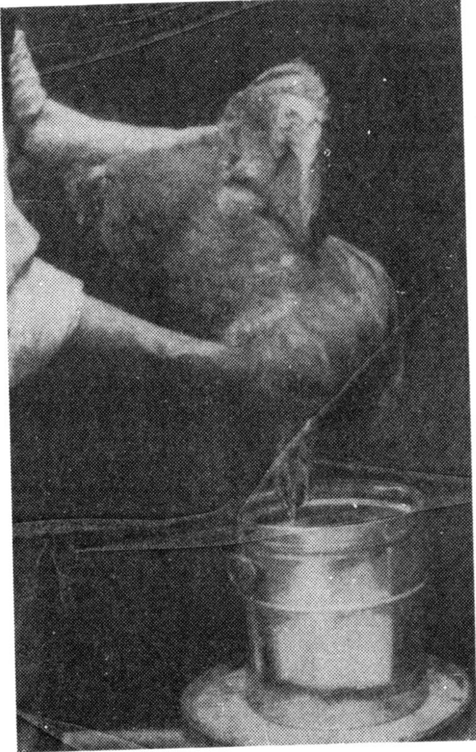

Fig. 2: Dipping the legs of a chicken in crude petroleum to control the scaly-leg mite.

near the base of the feathers; as a result, the feathers are often pulled or broken by the fowls. The mite, called the depluming mite, is very small, scarcely visible to the unaided eye and it is usually found in the follicles at the base of the feathers, particularly on the back and sides.

At times the mites leave their burrows and crawl about and this enables them to spread when chickens are in close contact.

The depluming mite can be completely eliminated from the flock by thoroughly dipping every chicken on the premises in a sulfur bath. To accomplish this a tub should be nearly filled with tepid water, 2 ounces of fine sulfur (98 percent passing a 325 mesh sieve) and ½ ounce of laundry soap being added for each gallon. The fowls should be submerged and the feathers raised so as to wet them thoroughly. The head of each bird should be ducked quickly two or three times.

If lice are also present on the birds, it is advisable to add ¾ ounce (1 heaping tablespoonful) of sodium fluoride to each gallon of water.

Since the soapy water thoroughly wets the feathers, this treatment should be applied only on warm sunny days or in a heated building.

Chiggers (Red Bugs or Harvest Mites)

Chiggers (*Eutrombicula alfreddugesi*) attack human beings and also infest chickens. Normally these small reddish mites feed upon wild animals, birds, snakes and lizards. The adult chiggers are the brilliant red, velvety mites that are sometimes seen crawling on the ground. The mite is parasitic only in its first stage of development. It does not penetrate the skin, as is commonly believed, but attaches itself in much the same manner as does the tick. After a few days it becomes engorged and drops off, if it is not dislodged by scratching. During the period of attachment it injects a poisonous secretion that sets up a violent local irritation and itching. On fowls, chiggers are inclined to attach themselves in groups, mainly on the wings, breast and neck. Injury to grown fowls is not very apparent except for the local lesions where the chiggers are or have been attached. Young chickens, however, are very susceptible to chigger infestations and soon become droopy, refuse to eat and frequently die in a short time (Fig. 3).

Chiggers are most abundant in the Southern States, especially on heavy soils. They usually appear some time after warm weather begins and are active until frost.

Since chigger injury to young turkeys and chickens is severe, where, these parasites are abundant it is advisable to hatch the chicks early and, in case of late hatches, to keep the chicks out of the grass and weeds. Keeping vegetation closely cut in the poultry yards is helpful and infestations may also be reduced by dusting the chicken ranges with sulfur at the rate of about 50 pounds per acre.

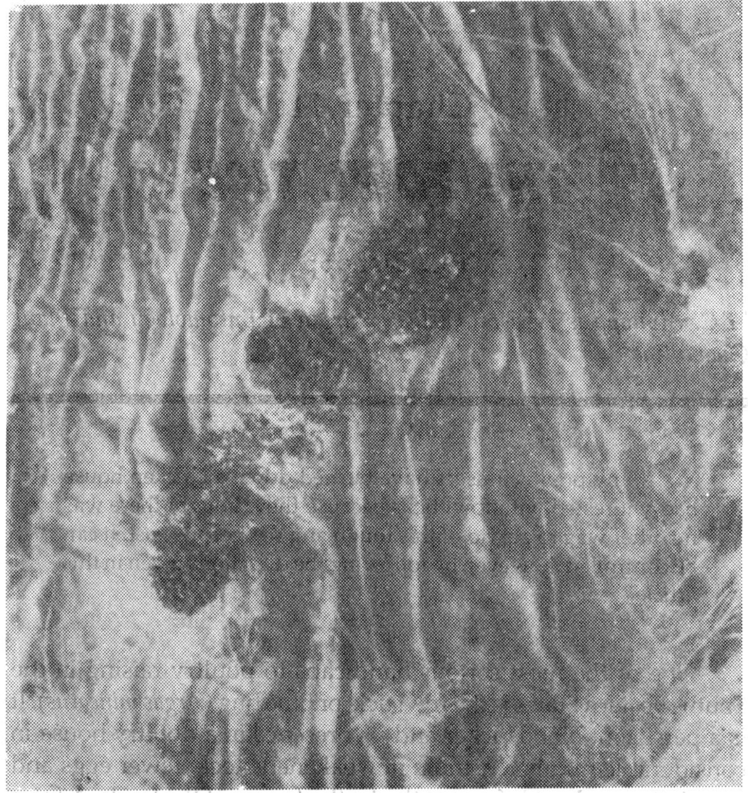

Fig. 3: Masses of chiggers on the skin of a chicken and the sores caused by them. Greatly enlarged.

Dusting the chicks lightly with sulfur also aids in protecting them. The lesions on grown chickens should be touched lightly with carbolated vaseline or sulfur ointment.

Chapter 11

THE FOWL TICK

F.C. Bishopp[1]

[1] *F.C. BiShopp is Assistant Chief, Bureau of Entomology and Plant Quarantine.*

Many poultry raisers have burned down a chicken house badly infested with fowl ticks because they thought there was no other way to get rid of this tough and dangerous pest. It can be controlled, however, by following the directions given in this article.

One of the most serious handicaps to poultry raising in the South-western States is the fowl tick, or blue bug (*Argas mineatus*). It is a persistent bloodsucker and its presence in a poultry house in considerable numbers results m weakened stock, fewer eggs and emaciation and not infrequently death of some of the fowls. A form of paralysis associated with this tick also affects many fowls, some of which die.

The tick was first found in southern Texas; it probably occurred in southern New Mexico, Arizona and California many years ago. More recently it has become established in Florida and it has spread northward in the South-western States so that it is now found in about two-thirds of California and Arizona and the south-western half of Oklahoma. Isolated infestations have occurred in Louisiana, Mississippi, Alabama, Nevada and Utah.

There is abundant opportunity for the tick to be shipped about the country because of its habit of remaining attached to fowls for several days and of hiding in crates and other places. If it were not for the adverse effect of cold and damp climates, it would no doubt by now have spread over the entire country.

Life History and Habits

The fowl tick is extremely hardy. It can withstand many insecticides and specimens have lived shut up in a small box without food for more than 3 years. In all its stages of development, the tick feeds exclusively on blood. Although it may occasionally bite domestic animals and human beings, it much prefers to feed on birds, including poultry. Chickens and turkeys are most affected, but ducks, geese and other domestic fowls, as well as some wild birds such as turkeys, quail, hawks and vultures are also attacked.

The tick is oval and very flat and has a leathery skin, so that it can easily hide in cracks. Its habits are also admirably adapted to those of the poultry on which it feeds. The hungry ticks become active at night and crawl about, seeking the fowls on the roost. The adults and those in the second, or nymphal, stages crawl onto the sleeping fowls and insert their beaks, drawing blood rapidly. Before day breaks they have returned to their hiding places in cracks about the roosts, walls and nests.

Mating takes place in the hiding places and a few days after feeding the female lays a batch of 50 to 100 brownish eggs (Fig. 1). Another blood meal is taken a few weeks later and a second clutch of eggs is deposited. This process may be repeated as many as 8 times and a total of 900 eggs may be deposited. During warm weather the eggs hatch in 10 or 12 days, but in cool weather the period may be as long as 3 months.

The young seed ticks that hatch from the eggs are grayish in colour and have six legs. After a few nights they crawl about actively in search of a fowl. When one is encountered they crawl upon it and attach themselves to various parts of the body, particularly where the feathers are sparse (Fig. 2). Over a period of 3 to 10 days the seed ticks enlarge considerably and become dark reddish blue. They leave the fowls at night and crawl about in search of cracks or crevices, or even rough places on the roosts in which to hide. During a period of 4 to 9 days spent in these hiding places, the seed ticks shed their skins, acquire another pair of legs and increase somewhat in size, although they remain very flat. A blood meal is taken in a few days

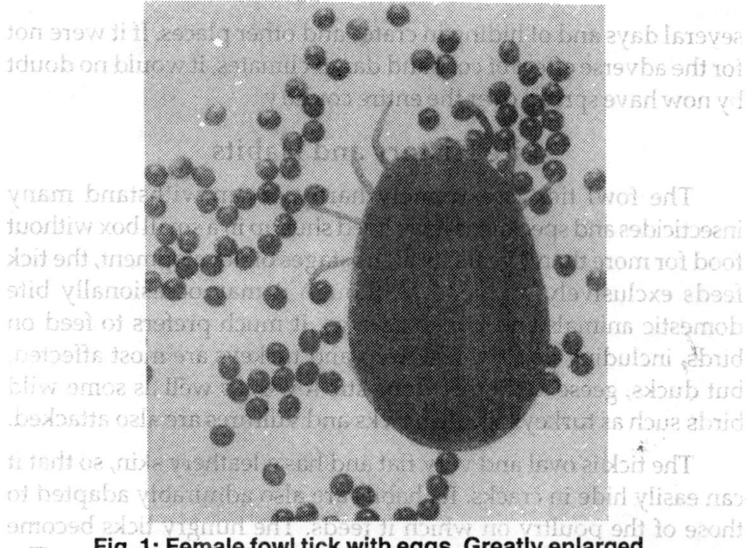

Fig. 1: Female fowl tick with eggs. Greatly enlarged.

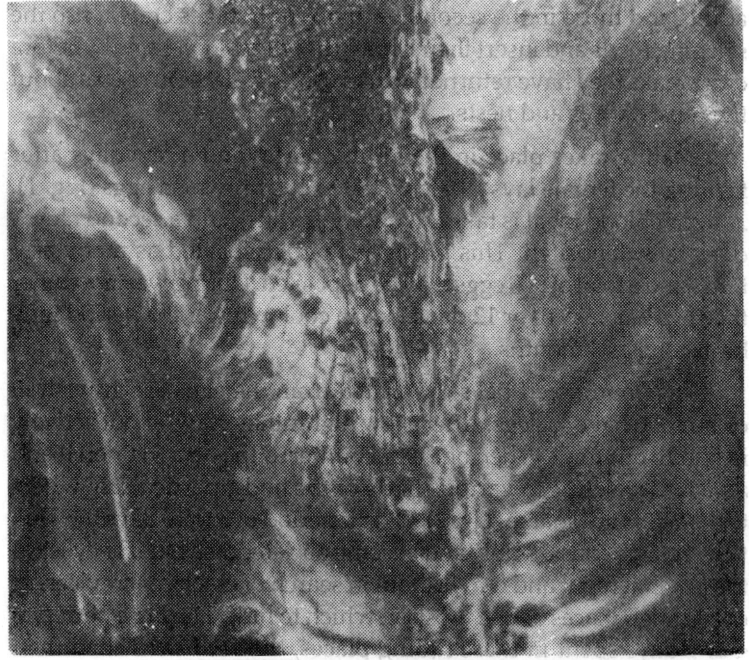

Fig. 2: The fowl tick. A mass of seed ticks (first stage) attached beneath wing of a chicken.

and then a second molt occurs, followed by another feeding and a molt to the adult stage. While hiding, the ticks move about to some extent, even when not hungry. They void a dark coloured excrement that dries on the wood and readily shows their presence.

Methods of Control

The great resistance of the fowl tick to insecticides makes it inadvisable to attempt to destroy the seed ticks on the fowls. Moreover, most of the ticks present at anyone time are to be found in the cracks and crevices around the roosts and roost supports, in the nest boxes and on adjacent walls. In old and heavy infestations the ticks are established throughout the poultry house, including the roof and not infrequently they are in barns and other outbuildings and in trees frequented by poultry.

To destroy these tough and well-hidden parasites a strong and penetrating material is required. Pure carbolineums, chemically known, as anthracene oil, are the most effective of the many materials tried. They are very penetrating and are so deadly that ticks placed on roosts painted with one of the carbolineums several weeks before gradually died off without laying eggs.

Crude petroleum and creosote oil are also useful in combating the fowl tick, but they are not as satisfactory in all respects as the carbolineums.

Treatment of Infested Buildings

In the morning remove the roosts, nests and any loose boards. In case of heavy infestations it is necessary to treat the entire inside of the chicken house. This is best done by spraying with a good bucket spray pump with a 10 or 12 foot lead of sound hose firmly attached and a cyclone or bordeaux nozzle.

The carbolineums and crude petroleum spray better if diluted with kerosene, 2 parts of the former to 1 part of the latter. If creosote oil is used, it should not be diluted. The spray should be driven into all cracks and crevices about the roosts, nests and walls. The roosts and nest boxes and the floor should then be sprayed. After the former are dry they may be put up again and fresh straw may be placed in the nests. Care should be taken by the operator not to get any of the material in his eyes or an unnecessary amount on his skin. The fowls should be kept out of the house until the material has soaked in and dried.

It is a common practice for poultry owners to shut the fowls out of a chicken house infested with fowl ticks. This should not be done, since it merely makes the birds roost in other places and thus scatter the infestation.

Usually one thorough spraying will clean out an infestation, but if it is scattered or very heavy, or if the house is double-walled, a second application 20 to 30 days after the first is required and in some instances a third has been found necessary.

If roosts and nests are built as described below, the second and third applications can be made with a brush, as it is seldom necessary to treat the roof and upper walls a second time if the roosts and nests are kept well covered with the oil.

Roost and Nest Construction

Roosts and nests should be as free from hiding places for the ticks as possible and should be so made that they can be easily examined and treated. Since the ticks tend to crawl upward rather than onto the ground, it has been found possible to largely protect fowls from attack by constructing the roosts on supports resting on the floor or driven into the ground. A convenient method is to notch the tops of the four supporting posts to receive a horizontal 2 by 4, which in turn is notched to receive the roosts. The roosts and their supports should be left without nailing, so that they may be easily lifted up and treated, None of the roost structure should be in contact with the wall. Where roosts are hinged to the back wall, as is often the case, the parts reaching the wall should be kept thoroughly treated with one of the materials mentioned.

Nest boxes may also be kept away from the walls and should be so constructed that they can be easily removed and treated, as shown in Fig. 3.

Cost of Medicines

Many chicken houses have been burned by their owners because of the prevalent idea that fowl ticks cannot be destroyed otherwise. The treatment described is not prohibitive in cost and its efficacy is attested by thousands of farmers and poultrymen.

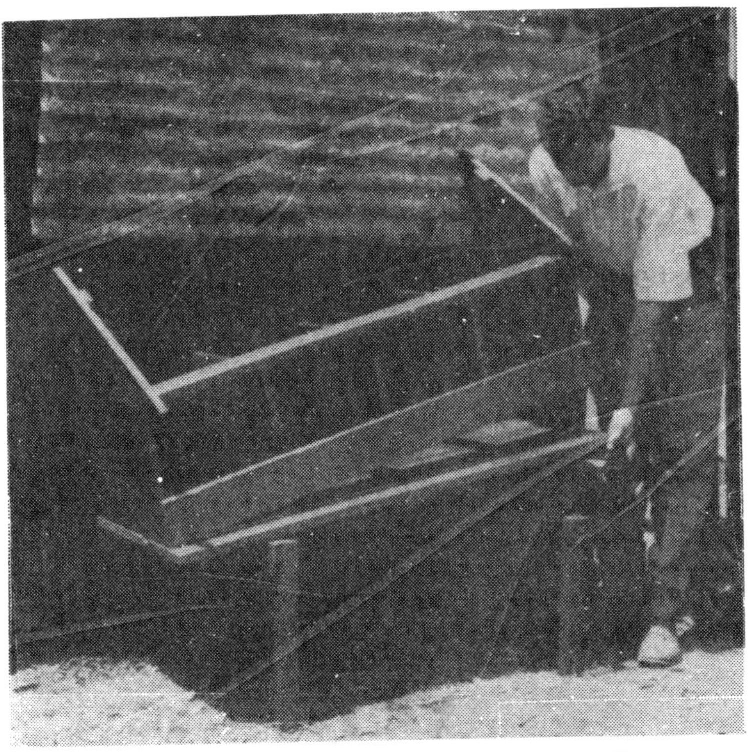

Fig. 3: Nest boxes so constructed as to be easily removed and treated.

A bucket pump is almost a necessity on any farm for spraying trees and applying whitewash. It usually costs from $3 to $8. The carbolineums usually cost from $1 to $1.50 a gallon, creosote oil 50 to 75 cents a gallon and crude petroleum 10 to 50 cents a gallon, according to the distance from the source of supply. A chicken house 10 by 14 feet would require 5 or 6 gallons of the mixture described. In a small house brush treatments of the roosts and nests would require less than 1 gallon.

Preventive Methods

It is much easier to keep ticks off uninfested premises than to eradicate an infestation. In starting in the poultry business, a site well removed from other flocks should be chosen and in arranging and constructing the building and pens the importance of the fowl tick and other poultry pests should be kept constantly in mind.

It is well to start with chicks from a hatchery known to be free of ticks and not to bring any grown fowls or used crates onto the premises. Any fowls brought in should be kept isolated for 10 days and the pen or coop containing them should be thoroughly sprayed. The methods described for combating the fowl tick are effective in controlling the common chicken mite, the bedbug and the Mexican chicken bug.

Chapter 12

BEDBUGS AS PESTS OF POULTRY

E.A. Back & F.C. Bishopp[1]

[1] *E.A. Back is Principal Entomologist of the Division of Insects Affecting Man and Animals and F.C. Bishopp is Assistant Chief, Bureau of Entomology and Plant Quarantine.*

The bedbug of human habitations is a much more common pest of poultry than most people realize. This article describes its habits and tells how to get rid of it in poultry plants.

Very few persons realize that bedbugs, which are so troublesome to human beings, also feed on other warm-blooded animals such as poultry. Frequently bedbugs get established in poultry and pigeon houses and they are often abundant in crates, both of wood and metal, in which poultry are shipped or in which they are held and fed at markets. As many as 2,500 well-grown, well-fed bedbugs were removed from the cracks of two wooden crates taken at random from one poultry market, no count being made of the a multitude of eggs and very young bedbugs present. As infestations progress, the cracks may become filled with egg-shells, molted skins and dead insects, all fused into a more or less solid mass by bedbug excrement. Fig. 1 is a photograph of such a crack filled with bedbugs and it shows the surrounding wood stained with many black specks. These specks, which are the most easily observable evidence of bedbug infestation, are the dried remains of the insects' semiliquid excrement.

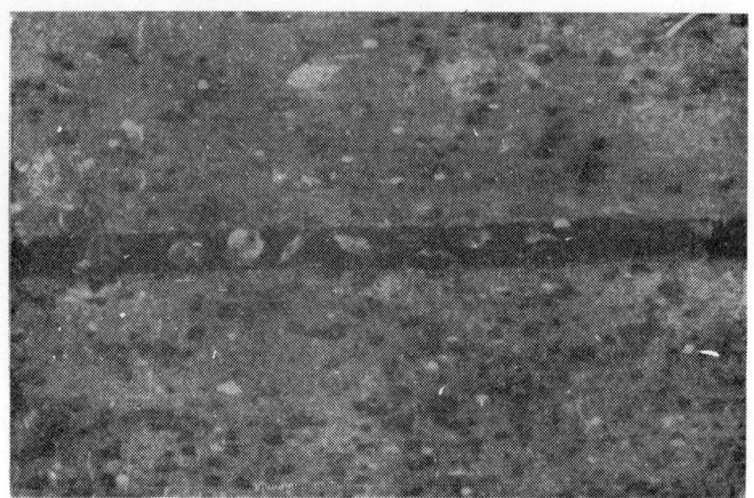

Fig. 1: Portion of a wooden poultry-shipping crate enlarged two diameters to show bedbugs crowded in a crack and black stains on wood formed by the drying of semi-liquid bedbug excrement.

Log houses, used for poultry on farms in many parts of the country, are especially subject to infestation by bedbugs, the cracks and the holes made by wood-boring insects in the logs making excellent retreats for the insects and giving protection not only against adverse weather but also against insecticides.

A mature, well-grown bedbug[2] is a wingless brown insect between one-fourth and three-eighths of an inch long. It is paper-thin when starved, but when engorged with blood it assumes the shape of the bugs shown in Fig. 2. It has a strong, characteristic odor.

Bedbugs are sucking insects. Their mouth parts are modified to form an elongated sharp beak, or proboscis, which can be thrust into the skin and through which blood can be drawn. It takes 3 to 5 minutes for a well-grown bedbug to become engorged with blood if

---

[2] BACK, E.A. BEDBUDGS. U.S. Dept. Agr. Leaflet 146, 8 pp., illus. 1937.

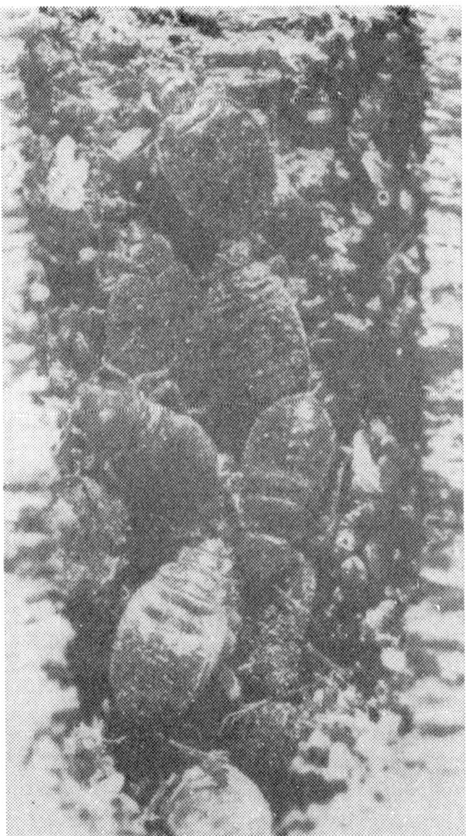

Fig. 2: Bedbugs, mostly well-fed, shown, greatly enlarged, in a spindle bole in a wooden crate three-eighths of an inch in diameter by eleven-sixteenths inch deep.

its feeding is unmolested. Once filled to capacity, the bug withdraws its beak and quickly crawls to its hiding place, where it remains for several days digesting its meal. When hunger finally re-asserts itself, the bed bug seeks a host for another meal.

Bedbugs normally feed at night or in subdued light. They are not known to carry any disease of poultry, but when allowed to become very abundant in hen houses or in crates in which chickens are held for fattening, they take so much blood that the chickens do not fatten, egg laying is reduced and setting hens may become weak or even die. When bedbugs become abundant in pigeon lofts, the effect on young squabs may be disastrous. According to Levi[3] the squabs from 1 to 3 days old become very anemic and, if the attack continues, die about the fourth day. The older squabs arid adult birds also become pale. The latter are restless and brooding is interfered with. The presence of bedbugs in poultry establishments is also a menace to the homes of people working in such places, as stray bedbugs are apt to be carried about on clothing and may establish infestations in furniture or bedding.

The mature female bedbug, under favorable conditions, lives from 6 to 10 months and may lay as many as 541 eggs, although 200 eggs is probably a fair average. The eggs are pearly white and about one thirty second of an inch long. They are deposited singly or in clusters in the crevices where bedbugs congregate. No eggs are laid when the temperature is lower than 50°F. and very few between 50° and 60°; maximum egg laying occurs only when the temperature is above 70° and when the female has ample opportunity to feed. Starved females soon stop laying eggs. At 70° F. or above, eggs hatch in 6 to 17 days, but at lower temperatures they may require 28 days.

The newly hatched, translucent, nearly colourless. young bedbug feeds at the first opportunity. During growth it resembles the parent. It molts, or sheds its skin, five times before reaching maturity. The cast skins are white and fluffy. Development from hatching to the adult stage requires 4 to 6 weeks during warm summer weather or in heated rooms. There may be three or four generations or even more in a year, depending on circumstances. In unheated poultry houses the bedbug overwinters mostly in the adult form. The older bedbugs commonly go 2 weeks to 2 months without food. Because bedbugs can subsist on the blood of mice and rats as well as that of poultry, human beings and domestic animals, the insect has been credited with living without food for periods of well over a year. It is a mystery to many poultry dealers how bedbugs can live over the winter in chicken crates used only during the summer and fall months, but usually the period of disuse is well within the capacity of the insects to exist under starvation conditions.

---

[3] LEVI, WENDELL MICTHELL. THE PIEGON. 512 pp., illus. Columbia, S.C. 1941.

The Mexican Chicken Bug and Related Forms

The Mexican chicken bug, or coruco (*Haematosiphon inodora*), is an important enemy of poultry in the semi-arid and arid Southwest. It is particularly abundant in adobe chicken houses and for this reason it is called the adobe bug locally. The chicken bug resembles the bedbug and its habits are similar, but it does not have characteristic bedbug odor.

Several species of bugs related to the bedbug and chicken bug are commonly associated with bats and swallows. Although swallows are frequently accused of bringing bugs into poultry establishments, this is probably an unusual occurrence, as the kind of bug found in swallows' nests is rarely found in poultry houses.

Control Methods

Control of bedbugs and chicken bugs in poultry establishments requires vigilance and persistent effort. Often these pests are overlooked until they are so numerous and widespread in the plant or about the farm buildings that it is difficult to eliminate them.

The bugs and their eggs are not difficult to kill when they can be reached with insecticidal sprays. Every effort should be made, therefore, to eliminate hiding places. Unnecessary boards and trash should be removed and when it is practicable cracks and holes should be filled with plaster, putty, or other materials. Roosts, nests, feeding batteries and other equipment should be simple in construction and easily moved for examination and treatment.

Bugs can be killed with fumigants, such as sulfur (3 pounds burned per 1,000 cubic feet), but most poultry houses are not built tightly enough to hold the gas sufficiently long to give good results. In general, spraying with creosote oil or one of the carbolmeums, as advised for the control of the fowl tick, is satisfactory for the treatment of infested buildings and equipment. Usually two sprayings will eliminate an infestation from a chicken house built of wood. In the case of feeding establishments where the pests are continually reintroduced, it is good practice to spray all crates once a month. Kerosene or pyrethrum-kerosene fly sprays may be employed where the staining caused by creosotes would be objectionable. In any event, the sprays must be thoroughly driven into cracks and crevices.

Pigeon lofts may be treated in the same way, but eggs and squabs may be injured by being returned to treated nests even when new nesting material is supplied. Levi has successfully used live steam in his large commercial pigeon plant. The steam is forced into the lofts and the temperature held at 125° F. or higher for 1 or 2 hours. The building is closed as tightly as possible with tar paper and canvas before being steamed.

Chapter 13

THE PIGEON FLY

F.C. Bishopp[1]

[1] *F.C. Bishopp is Assistant Chief, Bureau of Entomology and Plant Quarantine.*

This persistent enemy of pigeons and their close relatives is not only a bloodsucker but a carrier of pigeon malaria. It can be effectively controlled by the simple methods here outlined.

The pigeon fly (*Pseudolynchia canariensis*) is of sufficient importance as a parasite to warrant the attention of those who raise pigeons as messenger in the military service, for food, for the study of diseases or of genetics, or simply as a hobby.

These peculiar, bloodsucking flied feed only upon pigeons or closely related birds and breed in association with them. The flies attack squabs soon after the latter hatch and live and move about with ease among the closely set feathers of the adult pigeons. The loss of blood and the irritation caused by the flies are distinctly injurious to both squabs and adult birds. The flies also transmit the organism *Haemoproteus columbae,* which causes pigeon malaria, serving as its intermediate host.

The Insect and Its Habits

The pigeon fly is slightly smaller than the common housefly, flat and brownish. It has a rounded abdomen, rather long wings and a stout beak (Fig. 1). Its flight is quick and erratic and it does not usually leave the birds and take wing unless it is considerably

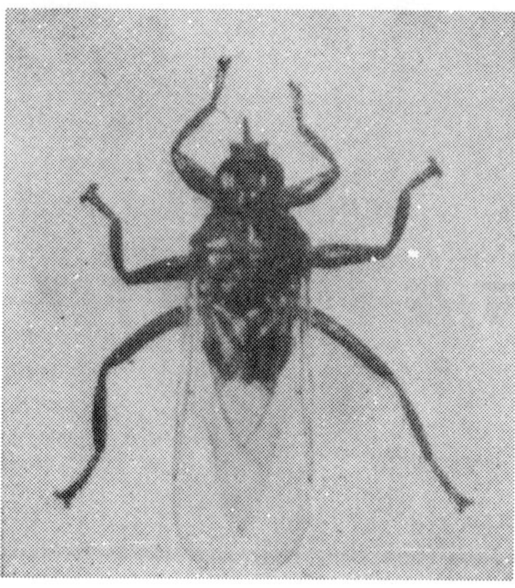

Fig. 1: The pigeon fly as seen from above. Enlarged about 6 times.

disturbed. When driven off the host, it usually alights on some nearby object, especially a moving object and in buildings it often goes toward the light at windows or open doors.

On grown pigeons the flies may be found on any part of the body. They crawl rapidly from place to place or on among the feathers, often moving backwards or sideways. Squabs often become heavily infested especially when they are partly feathered, the flies usually congregating at the base of the feathers of the tail and wings.

Both male and female flies suck blood. They leave no marked evidence of their bites on pigeons but evidently annoy them a great deal. They frequently bite human beings, especially where squabs are dressed for market and are often very annoying to the workers. The points of attack may continue to show signs of irritation for 4 or 5 days.

The flies are active on the pigeons throughout the winter in the warmer parts of the country, though their numbers diminish markedly toward spring. The insect has the peculiar habit of retaining its larvae until they have pupated. The fly gives birth to the ovoid pupae one at a time. The pupae are about one-eighth of an inch long, at first pale yellowish in colour but soon turning brownish and within about 3 hours becoming shiny black (Fig. 2). They are usually deposited while the flies are on the pigeons and may hang temporarily in the feathers, though they soon drop off among the nest material, where they usually fall through to the bottom of the nest boxes.

At an average temperature of 73° F. the pupal stage lasts 25 days during hot weather to 31 days or longer in cold weather.

The fly emerges by pushing open the front end of the hard pupa case, which splits along a definite line running around the case about one-third of its length from the head end, The fly is pale and soft at first, but it soon hardens, turns brown and is ready to take a meal of blood.

Methods of Control

Pigeons should be kept in confinement and the loft should be so arranged as to make it easy to clean the nests and floors. Probably the simplest and most effective single step in the control of pigeon flies is to clean out the nests thoroughly every 25 days. The pupae

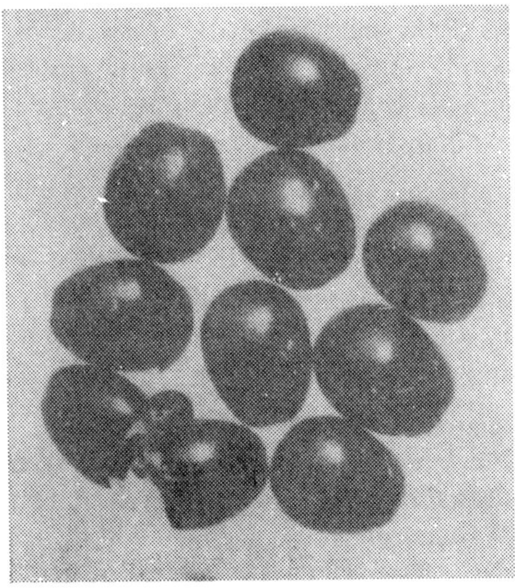

Fig. 2: Pupae of the pigeon fly. Enlarged about 6 times.

are so smooth and round that, as already indicated, they usually drop to the bottom of the nest boxes. This makes it possible to pick up the nest, brush the dirt and pupae off the bottom of the box and return the nest with little disturbance. Since the pupae roll freely, nest cleaning should proceed from the top downward and care should be taken to brush the pupae out of the cracks. It is well to spread a piece of canvas on the floor beneath the boxes before cleaning to catch any pupae that may drop to the floor. The trash may then be burned or, if used for fertilizer, stored in a screened pit or bin, preferably one in which there is a conical fly trap to catch the flies that emerge. Most of the pupae will be destroyed if the material is scattered on a field and promptly plowed under to a depth of 4 or 5 inches.

The pupae are rather resistant to insecticides, but they may be killed by being wetted thoroughly with a high-grade pyrethrum-kerosene fly spray.

A number of insecticides have been found to be effective in killing the flies on the birds. The main difficulty is to reach the insects and yet not burn the skin or stain the feathers of the pigeons. One of the most easily applied and effective treatments for squabs is fresh pyrethrum powder. From one to three pinches, depending on the size of the squab, dusted in the feather tufts, will kill all flies present. Grown pigeons are harder to treat and on them the powder is less effective, especially when the birds are flying about. Derris or cube powder, containing 3 to 5 percent rotenone, is nearly as effective as pyrethrum and should be used in the same way.

Kerosene, extract of pyrethrum, prepared and sold as high-grade fly spray, is very effective in killing the flies either free in handling and killing rooms or on the birds. The material is applied tightly on the birds in a fine spray as the feathers are lifted. This must be done very carefully, however, since an excessive amount, especially on squabs, will burn the skill and make the eyes sore.

Many lofts are free of pigeon flies and care should be taken to treat any new stock brought into a clean loft and to check closely on birds sent to races and shows. Special care should be taken to keep racing pigeons free from these flies and other parasites, which distinctly handicap the performance of the birds.

Cold weather apparently kills the pigeon flies in many lofts in the North and when this occurs an effort should be made to keep them fly-free during the summer, when the parasite can breed rather rapidly.

The control measures used against the pigeon fly are very helpful in keeping down other insect enemies of the pigeon.

Chapter 14

NUTRITIONAL DISEASES OF POULTRY

Harry W. Titus [1]

[1] *Harry, W. Titus is Senior Biological Chemist, in Charge of Poultry Nutrition Investigations, Animal Nutrition Division, Bureau of Animal Industry.*

This article discusses 16 well-defined nutritional disease, a group of less-well-defined diseases and the effect of nutritional deficiencies on growth and reproduction. The material is especially significant because a good deal of rather precise work has been done in this field with poultry.

A fairly large number of different elements and compounds are required for the normal nutrition of poultry. If one or more of them are not present in the diet in adequate quantity, or if certain ones are present in an unsuitable ratio, there is a disturbance of nutrition, or of the functioning of the body, which may be referred to as a nutritional disease. Other nutritional disease may result from harmful elements or compounds in the diet.

Knowledge in the filed of nutritional diseases of poultry is in a state of active change. That which is believed to be true today may be disproved tomorrow, or, as perhaps more often happens, may prove to be only part of the truth. In several instances an abnormal condition that was originally thought to be result of a single nutritional deficiency has been found to result from a multiple deficiency. A good example is polyneutritis in the chicken. At one time the case of this condition was believed to be a deficiency of vitamin B and this vitamin was–and still is–referred to as the antineuritic vitamin and was given the name "aneurin." It is now known that the condition originally described as polyneuritis gallinarum was produced by diets deficient in vitamins A, E and G and pantothenic acid as well as in vitamin B_1. Moreover, it has been shown that a deficiency of vitamin B_1 alone does not produce nerve degeneration in the chicken, although it does have other serious effects on the nerves.

Vitamin A Deficiency

If day-old chicks are placed on a diet markedly deficient in vitamin A, their rate of growth falls below normal after about 2 weeks and then declines rapidly. The first characteristic symptoms, other than the decrease in rate of growth, are droopiness, a staggering gait and a ruffled appearance of the feathers. These symptoms may appear as early as the end of the third week. Some of the chicks die before the end of the fourth week and most of the others before they are 5 weeks old. Growth usually ceases several days before death occurs. In many of the chicks that survive for more than a week after the first characteristic symptoms appear, the eyes become inflamed and there is a discharge from the nostrils; in some there are a swelling around the eyes and an accumulation of sticky exudate beneath the lods.

With a diet partially deficient in vitamin A, the first symptoms may not appear until the chicks are 5 or 6 weeks old. In this case, a larger proportion of the chicks eventually have inflamed eyes and an accumulation of white cheesy material under the lids (Fig. 1).

In mature chickens the symptoms develop much more slowly than in growing chicks, but the inflammation of the eyes becomes strikingly more pronounced. Often there are a white membranous film over the nictitating membrane, or third eyelid, and a cheesy exudate or discharge, in the conjunctival sacs. There may also be a sticky discharge, either clear or turbid, from the nostrils.

The symptoms of vitamin A deficiency in the turkey poult are in general similar to those in the chick, but according to Hinshaw and Lloyd (*21*)[2] the disease is much more acute in poults. These authors described the symptoms in poults that had received little or no

---

[2] Italic numbers in parentheses refer to Literature Cited.

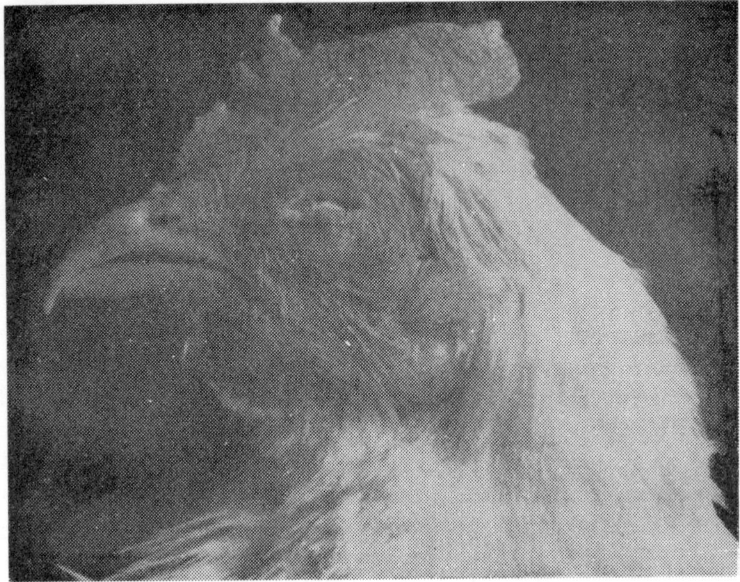

Fig. 1: Effects of vitamin A deficiency in an advanced stage. Note the swelling around the eye and the cheesy exudate under the lids. (Courtesy of J.R. Beach, Division of Veterinary Science, California Agricultural Experiment Station, Berkeley, Calif.)

vitamin A from the time of hatching as "those of an acute-infectio-contagious disease except that fever was absent." In chicks that were fed the same diet as the poults and kept in the same pen there was a marked nervousness, which the poults did not exhibit.

Findings After Death[3]

An examination of chickens and turkeys that die as a result of vitamin A deficiency reveals lesions, or tissue changes, in many parts of the body, their location and severity depending to some extent on the age of the bird, the degree of the deficiency and the

[3] In this article, material on post mortem findings and also material on diseases that seldom or never occur in ordinary poultry production but are of great interest from the experimental standpoint are set in smaller type.

length of time between the appearance of the first symptoms and death.

In mature birds lesions resembling pustules are almost invariably found in the mouth, pharynx and esophagus (Fig. 2); in young growing birds these are seen much less frequently. Usually there are white or grayish-white deposits of urates in the kidneys and ureters, which occur more frequently in the chick than in the poult. Sometimes there are deposits of urates on the surface of the heart, liver and spleen. Hinshaw and Lloyd (*21*) have reported that they found white, flaky, uratelike deposits between thickened folds of the bursa Fabricii in most of the poults and chicks they examined and Heywang and Morgan (*20*) have confirmed their findings in the case of the chick.

In general, there is a keratinization, or hornlike hardening, of the epithelial cells of the olfactory, respiratory, upper alimentary and urinary tracts, In severe cases, especially if the birds are mature, virtually every organ in the body may be affected. Also, there are degenerative changes in both the central and peripheral nervous

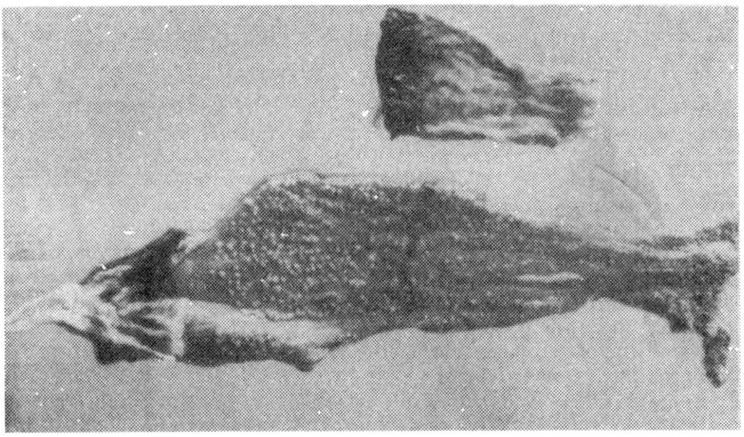

Fig. 2: Pustulelike lesions in the esophagus caused by vitamin A deficiency. (Courtesy of L.D. Bushnell, Bacteriology Department, Kansas Agricultural Experiment Station.)

systems and these explain the staggering gait, which is one of the first symptoms of vitamin A deficiency in chickens, and the extreme lack of muscular coordination in advanced cases.

Function of Vitamin A and Prevention of Deficiencies

Histological examinations–that is, examinations of the minute structure–of the tissues of chickens that have been fed a diet deficient in vitamin A indicate that one of the functions–if not the primary function–of vitamin A is the proper nourishment and repair of all the epithelial structures, external and internal, in the body. In extreme vitamin A deficiency in the chicken the uric acid content of the blood may increase to eight or nine times its normal value, The accumulation of uric acid in the blood and the previously mentioned occurrence of deposits of uric acid in the ureters, the kidneys and elsewhere are probably results of failure of repair of epithelial structures, especially those of the kidneys,

Studies made with other animals have shown that vitamin A is necessary for the normal functioning of the eyes. Apparently, however, it plays no detectable role in the absorption and metabolism of fats, carbohydrates and proteins.

Vitamin A has been referred to as the anti-infective vitamin, but repeated attempts to show that it affects the mechanisms that give the body immunity against infections have failed. When the diet is deficient in vitamin A, however, the epithelium, or, surface layer of the mucous membranes is damaged and as a result the entry of bacteria is made easier. Thus, although vitamin A is of no value in making an animal immune to infectious diseases, it is of value in maintaining the "first line of defense," the epithelial structures.

As has been pointed out by Barger and Card (2), a partial deficiency of vitamin A in diets for poultry is more common than is generally supposed. They state that it is especially likely to occur in regions where the summers are hot and dry and there is a resulting shortage of green forage. Partial Vitamin A deficiency is often an aftermath of drought. A partial vitamin A deficiency is also possible when flocks are closely confined unless an adequate supply is included in the feed.

The obvious method of preventing the development of vitamin A deficiency disease in poultry is to supply an adequate quantity of this vitamin in the feed. The minimum vitamin A requirement of the growing chick is about 675 to 775 International units per pound of feed; that of the growing poult is about 2½ times, as much. An adequate supply, as distinguished from the minimum, is about 1,450 International units per pound of feed for the chick and about 3,650 per pound of feed for the poult. The vitamin A in mixed feeds, however, is not very stable and for this reason it is a good practice to formulate the diets of chicks and poults so that they will contain 3,000 and 7,500 International units per pound of feed, respectively. The feed of chickens kept for egg production should contain approximately 3,150 International units per pound. The feed of breeding stock–chickens or turkeys–should contain about 4,720 units per pound.

The approximate vitamin A contents of some of the richer sources of this vitamin used in feeding poultry are as follows:

	International units per pound
Fortified cod-liver oil	1,360,770
Fortified sardine oil	1,360,770
Cod-liver oil	385,550
Sardine oil	52,000
Alfalfa-leaf meal, dehydrated	95,000
Alfalfa-leaf meal	32,000
Alfalfa meal	13,000
Corn-gluten meal	6,800
Yellow corn	3,180

Vitamin B_1 Deficiency

The symptoms of vitamin B_1 deficiency are similar in chickens and turkeys and are essentially the same at different ages. A diet containing little or no vitamin B_1 but otherwise adequate causes a prompt decrease in appetite, followed soon by a steady decline in live weight. After 7 to 10 days there is progressive development of general paralysis. The extensor muscles of the legs are the first to become affected, but soon the paralysis extends to the wings and neck and, finally to all the muscles. In the early stages of paralysis the bird swallows feed or water with great difficulty; in the later stages the body temperature falls and the head is raised and drawn back. Death follows, usually within 1 or 2 days after the typical symptom of head retraction appears (Fig 3).

When the diet is only partially deficient in vitamin B_1, 30 days or more may elapse before the symptoms of paralysis appear. In the ability of chickens and other birds to survive on diets that are only partially deficient in vitamin B_1 there are marked individual differences. In adult and nearly grown birds there is a loss of about 20 percent of the initial live weight before death occurs. .

The first symptom in pigeons is a partial loss of the ability to walk. The next symptom is uncontrolled movement of the head. Finally, head retraction occurs and the legs are drawn up close to the body; often the bird turns somersaults. As in the chicken, death follows soon after head retraction occurs.

Findings After Death

With few exceptions, the diets that have been used in studying vitamin B_1 deficiency have not contained adequate quantities of some

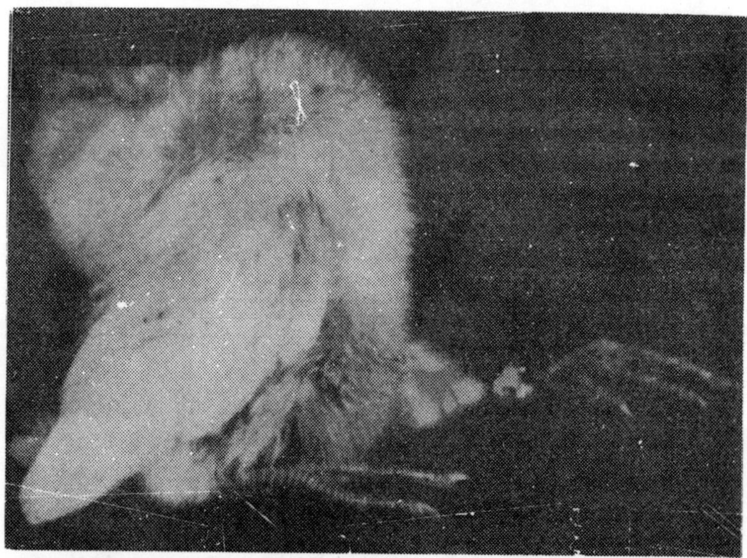

Fig. 3: Head retraction is a characteristic symptom of vitamin B_1 deficiency in the late stage. (Courtesy of L.C. Norris, Nutrition Division, Department of Poultry Husbandry, Cornell University.)

of the other vitamins, especially vitamin A and those that commonly occur with vitamin B_1 in natural products. As a matter of fact, the diets that were used in the first studies of vitamin B_1 deficiency in the chicken and pigeon were also markedly deficient in vitamin A. Many of the earlier descriptions of the findings after death from what was considered to be vitamin B_1 deficiency were for this reason in reality descriptions of the results of a multiple deficiency.

For many years it was believed that a deficiency of vitamin B_1 caused extensive degeneration of the peripheral nervous system. Engel and Phillips (*11*) have shown, however, that there is no nerve degeneration in either the rat or the chick when the vitamin-B_1-deficient diet contains a fully adequate supply of vitamin A and vitamin G. Moreover, there is evidence that the withholding of feed produces in the chicken and other animals many of the changes that are observed when a diet deficient in vitamin B_1 is fed.

At the time this is being written there is not available to the writer a good description of the post mortem findings in birds that have died as a result of an uncomplicated vitamin B_1 deficiency.

Function of Vitamin B_1 and Prevention of Deficiencies

According to the evidence now available, vitamin B_1 is required for the proper metabolism of carbohydrates.[4]

Nitzescu and Ioanid (*39*) found that it hens are deprived of vitamin B_1 the sugar content of their blood decreases and remains below normal for 10 to 14 days, then rises rapidly in the next few days to more than twice normal. If vitamin B_1 is injected, the sugar content of the blood returns to normal. They found also that injections of vitamin B_1 produce appreciable decreases in the sugar content of the blood of normal hens.

The animal has relatively little capacity for storing vitamin B_1 and for this reason, when there is a multiple deficiency of this and other vitamins, the symptoms of vitamin B_1 deficiency tend to appear first. That these symptoms, paralysis and head retraction–the first

[4] More specifically soon after vitamin B_1 is absorbed from the Intestinal tract, it is converted into cocarboxylase, which functions as a coenzyme in the metabolism of pyruvic acid. When the diet does not contain enough vitamin B_1, pyruvic acid accumulates in various tissues of the body and exerts a toxic effect on the nervous system.

except cessation of growth–are the result of vitamin B_1 deficiency may be shown conclusively by causing them to disappear in a short time–often less than 2 hours-by the administration of synthetic crystalline vitamin B_1. That these symptoms can thus be made to disappear is evidence that they are not the result of nerve degeneration.

Vitamin B_1 deficiency in poultry is rarely observed under practical conditions. It can be produced by feeding a diet that consists wholly of polished rice or degerminated grain or specially formulated diets.

In practical poultry production no special precautions need be taken to prevent vitamin B_1 deficiency. The minimum vitamin B_1 requirement of poultry is about 90 to 135 International units per pound of feed. An adequate supply is about 180 International units per pound of feed. Most diets for poultry contain two to three times this quantity.

The approximate vitamin B_1 contents of some of its richer sources in feeding poultry are as follows:

	International units per pound
Yeast, brewers, dried	4,500
Soybean meal	1,600
Oats	1,200
Wheat middlings, standard	1,000
Wheat bran	840
Wheat	680
Skim milk, dried	500
Buttermilk, dried	450
Barley	400
Corn	400

Vitamin B_6 Deficiency

Very little is known about the vitamin B_6 requirements of poultry or the symptoms of vitamin B_6 deficiency. In 1939 Jukes (23) reported that the symptoms in chicks consist of slow growth, depressed appetite and inefficient utilization of feed, followed in some cases by spasmodic convulsions and death, but in 1940 he reported (*24*) that the diet that he had used in studying vitamin B_6 deficiency was deficient even when supplemented with the vitamin. More recently, Hegsted, Oleson, Elvehjem and Bart (*19*) reported that the only symptoms of vitamin B_6 deficiency that they had observed in growing chicks were lack of growth and extreme weakness.

Vitamin B_6 is widely distributed in nature and for this reason a deficiency does not occur among poultry that are fed practical diets but would be produced only by special, highly simplified diets. Yeast, wheat germ and egg yolk are some of the best sources of B_6 vitamin; other good sources are kidney, liver, fish meal, dried skim milk, dried buttermilk, alfalfa products and rice polishings; all the grains appear to be fairly good sources.

Vitamin D Deficiency and Rickets

Abnormal development of the bones of growing chickens, turkeys and other kinds of poultry may result from a number of dietary, causes, among which are:

(1) A deficiency of one or more of the following substances: Vitamin D, calcium, phosphorus, manganese and choline;

(2) A marked unbalance of calcium and phosphorus; and

(3) The presence of certain substances that make the vitamin D or the phosphorus unavailable.

The discussion here is restricted to those conditions in which the absorption and metabolism of vitamin D, calcium and phosphorus are directly involved. The condition that results from a deficiency of manganese or choline or both is discussed later.

Some writers–for example McGowan and Emslie (*34*)–distinguish between rickets and another condition of the bones, osteoporosis, on the ground that the former is the result of a deficiency of phosphorus and the latter of a deficiency of calcium. The distinction is warranted because the changes that occur in the bones are not the same in the two conditions. However, both may be prevented or cured by including sufficient vitamin D in the diet, unless the deficiency of phosphorus or calcium is very marked.

At the time of hatching, the chick is essentially osteoporotic, that is, its bones have a such lower calcium-phosphorus ratio than they do later on; hence it requires an immediate supply of calcium in its diet. If the diet is deficient in calcium or if that which is present is unavailable as a result of a deficiency of vitamin D, the osteoporotic condition becomes more pronounced. If there is an adequate supply of calcium but a deficiency of phosphorus or vitamin D or both, rickets develops.

Rickets may be produced on diets that contain adequate quantities of vitamin D, calcium and phosphorus if the diets also contain large quantities of certain inorganic compounds, such as soluble salts of iron, lead and beryllium. This is because iron, lead and beryllium form insoluble compounds with the phosphorus and make it unavailable. Excessive quantities of calcium in the diet of growing chicks may also make much of the phosphorus unavailable as a result of the formation of the relatively insoluble calcium phosphate. A diet deficient in vitamin D is therefore more rachitogenic (rickets-causing) if it contains an excessive quantity of calcium than if it contains a much smaller but adequate quantity.

A condition called sulfur rickets may result from the inclusion in the diet of 2 percent or more of sulfur for the control of coccidiosis. If the particles of sulfur are very small (for example, colloidal), less than 2 percent may cause this condition. Why sulfur has this effect is not known, but there are reasons for believing that it interferes with the absorption of vitamin D. The condition is relieved but not entirely eliminated by doubling or trebling the vitamin D content of the diet. Sunshine appears to be more effective, than vitamin D in preventing sulfur rickets.

The rickety and osteoporotic conditions encountered in the practical production of poultry are most frequently caused by a deficiency of vitamin D rather than by a deficiency of calcium or phosphorus or the presence in the diet of large quantities of soluble salts of iron, beryllium, or lead.

If a vitamin D-deficient diet is fed, beginning with the first feeding, the first symptoms usually make their appearance in the poult toward the end of the third week and in the chick about a week later. Usually most of the poults die within 5 weeks and a large proportion of the chicks within 8 weeks.

In the adult chicken the first symptom of vitamin D deficiency is a thinning of the shells of its eggs. If the deficiency is marked, there is a fairly prompt decrease in both egg production and hatchability. After a time the breast bones become distinctly less rigid. Adult chickens, however, can live for months on a diet that supplies practically no vitamin D.

The first symptoms of vitamin D deficiency in the growing chicken and turkey are a tendency to rest frequently in a squatting position, a disinclination to walk and a lame, stiff-legged gait. These symptoms are readily distinguishable from those of vitamin A deficiency in that in vitamin D deficiency the chick or poult at first is alert rather than droopy and walks with a lame rather than a staggering gait. Other symptoms, in the usual order of their occurrence, are retardation of growth, enlargement of the hock joints, beading at the ends of the ribs and marked softening of the beak (Fig. 4). As in many other nutritional diseases of poultry, the feathers soon acquire a ruffled appearance.

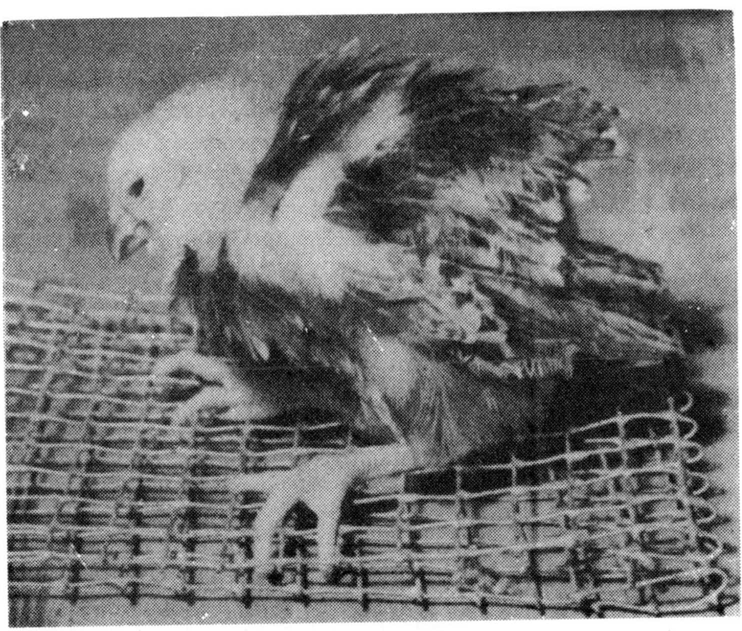

Fig. 4: Vitamin D deficiency in a young chicken. Note the crossed beak, which is soft and rubbery, and the inability to stand.

Gross Changes and Chemical Findings

In the chick and poult, vitamin D deficiency produces marked changes in the, bones and the parathyroid and thyroid glands and variable changes in the calcium and phosphorus content of he blood. The bones may be soft or only moderately so, but in any case their ash (mineral) content is much less than normal and in some instances the ash content of the tibia (drumstick bones) may be as little as 27 percent on a moisture-and-fat-free basis. (The normal ash value for the tibiae of young chicks is about 46 percent). The epiphyses, or growing ends, of the long bones are usually enlarged. The parathyroid becomes enlarged, sometimes to eight times its normal size, as a result of an increase in both the size of the cells and the number of epithelial cells. At must there is no great change in the size of the thyroid, but there is an appreciable increase in the number of cells.

The changes in the calcium and phosphorus content of the blood depend on the calcium and phosphorus content of the diet. If the diet has a high calcium content, the calcium content of the blood may be approximately normal and the phosphorus content low. In such a case the bones may be somewhat rarefied, rather than soft. If there is a deficiency of both calcium and phosphorus in the diet, the blood may contain less than the normal quantities of these elements. When there is a deficiency of phosphorus, the bones tend to be soft and may be bent.

In adult chickens a deficiency of vitamin D eventually produces changes in the parathyroid similar to those produced in chicks. The bones tend to become rarefied (osteoporotic) rather than soft.

Function of Vitamin D and Prevention of Deficiencies

It must be concluded that vitamin D is required for the normal metabolism of calcium and phosphorus in the chicken, but the exact manner in which it performs its function is not known. A diet deficient in vitamin D does not produce rickets in rats if it contains suitable quantities of calcium and phosphorus, but rickets is, always produce in chickens by a deficiency of vitamin D, even when the diet contains calcium and phosphorus in suitable quantities. There is good evidence that in the rat vitamin D regulates the absorption of calcium and phosphorus from the intestine and it is highly probable that it performs the same function in the chicken.

Before the discovery of the importance of vitamin D in the nutrition of poultry, it was not possible to raise poultry in strict confinement; that is, without access to sunshine. Even under normal conditions, rickets was likely to occur in poultry whenever there were long periods of cloudy or rainy weather during the brooding season. It is now a common practice to include at least some vitamin D in the diet of poultry whether they have access to sunshine or not. Even so, rickets is occasionally encountered as a result of usiug an inferior grade of cod-liver oil or other source of vitamin D.

Laying flocks are frequently housed in quarters into which little or no sunshine penetrates and many such flocks suffer from the effects of vitamin D deficiency. Even when laying flocks are allowed to range the year round, they may get too little sunshine during the late fall, winter and early spring. It is advisable, therefore, to include some vitamin D in the diet of all laying stock, whether or pot they are allowed to range.

The usual sources of vitamin D, other than sunshine, are cod-liver oil, sardine oil, certain other fish oils and "D"-activated animal sterol. Vitamin D deficiency is readily prevented or cured by a suitable quantity of any one of those materials. The minimum vitamin D requirement of the growing chick is about 60 to 90 A.O.A.C. chick units[5] per pound of feed; that of the growing poult is about 2 to 3% times as much. An adequate supply for the chick, is about 180 A.O.A.C. chick units per pound of feed and for the poult about 360 units. The duckling apparently requires about as much vitamin D as the poult.

Chickens that are being kept for the eggs they produce should receive about 360 A.O.A.C. chick units of vitamin D per pound of feed and breeding stock–both chickens and turkeys–about 540 units.

Cod-liver oil that is sold as such in interstate commerce is required by law to contain not less than 85 United States Pharmacopoeia units of vitamin D per gram, or about 38,560 U.S.P. units per pound. In the case of cod-liver oil 1 U.S.P. unit of vitamin D is equal to 1 A.O.A.C. chick unit. The fortified cod-liver oil and sardine oils now on the market are usually guaranteed to contain about 181,600 A.O.A.C. chick units per pound. Other oils and other

[5] The standard unit of the Association of Official Agricultural Chemists.

products used as sources of vitamin D in feeding poultry are usually sold on the basis of a guaranteed number of A.O.A.C. chick units, per gram or per pound.

Vitamin E Deficiency

By feeding a diet high in fat but markedly deficient in vitamin E to chicks, ducklings and poults, Pappenheimer, Goettsch and Jungherr (*41*) produced nutritional encephalomalacia (crazy-chick disease) in the chicks, nutritional myopathy (a disease of the muscles), in the ducklings and nutritional myopathy of the gizzard in the poults. They were able to prevent or at least greatly reduce the incidence of the encephalomalacia in the chicks by including various vegetable oils in their diet. They completely prevented the development of encephalomalacia by administering small quantities of alpha-tocopherol (vitamin E) by mouth. In a single experiment with ducklings the nutritional myopathy was prevented by substituting 5 percent of hydrogenated cottonseed oil for an equal weight of lard in the diet. In the case of poults the administration by mouth of 0.34 cubic centimeter of wheat-germ oil per head per day in gelatin capsules greatly reduced the incidence of the gizzard condition but did not eliminate it completely.

Symptoms of Nutritional Encephalomalacia in the Chick

When a diet such as that used by Pappenheimer and associates (*41*) is fed to day-old chicks, the encephalomalacia may occur as early as the seventh and as late as the fifty-sixth day, but the highest incidence is between the fifteenth and thirtieth days after hatching. The average age at which the disease occurs is about 5 weeks. In older chicks the average number of days before the onset of the disease depends on the age at which the deficient diet is first fed; the older the chicks are, up to 8 weeks of age, the more quickly they are affected. The disease rarely occurs among chicks more than 8 weeks old.

The symptoms of nutritional encephalomalacia are described very well by its popular name, "crazy-chick disease." When the chicks attempt to walk, they often fall forward, backward, or to one side and then wheel in circles. In advanced cases there is frequently complete prostration, with the legs extended, the head sometimes retracted and tremors of both head and legs (Fig. 5).

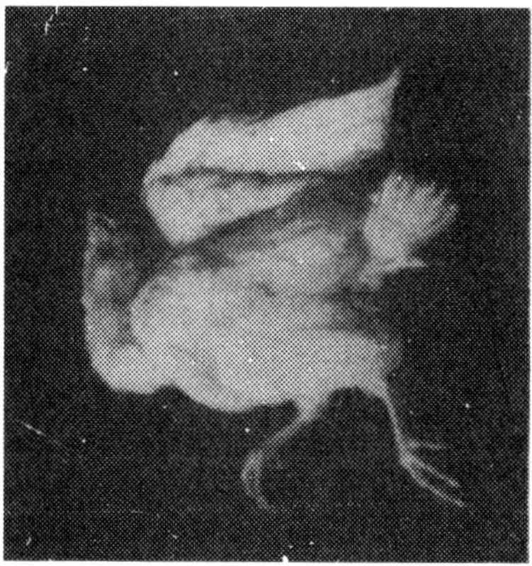

Fig. 5: A chicken prostrated by nutritional encephalomalacia, or crazy-chick disease, in an advanced stage. The retracted head is also a result of vitamin E deficiency. (Courtesy of Erwin Jungherr, Department of Animal Disease, Storrs Agricultural Experiment Station, Storrs, Conn).

Extensive lesions are usually found in the brains of chicks that have died of nutritional encephalomalacia. The cerebellum (the hind part of the brain) is most commonly affected; but in somewhat more than 25 percent of all cases lesions are found also in the cerebral hemispheres and in about 12 percent f of all cases in the medulla. In some cases four-fifths of the cerebellum may be affected and in others the lesions may be so small that they cannot be detected with the unaided eye. The affected tissues change from pink to greenish yellow and in the healing stage to a rusty brown. For a rather complete description of the microscopic changes that take place in the brain, the reader is referred to Pappenhelmer, Goettsch and Jungherr's monograph (*41*).

Symptoms of Nutritional Myopathy, or Muscle Disease

The symptoms of nutritional myopathy in ducklings appear quite suddenly, usually in the second or third week. In the early stages the ducklings walk awkwardly, with their feet turned in and sometimes overlapping. Often they are found sprawled out and unable to rise. Sometimes there are coarse tremors. Only the skeletal muscles show pathologic changes; the muscles are pale in colour–a light creamy yellow rather than dark red. There are widespread hyalme necrosis and some edema, or watery swelling.

When the Pappenheirner-Goettsch diet is fed to young poults, there are no specific outward indications that anything is wrong, but on post mortem examination, lesions or tissue changes are found in the muscular wall of the gizzard. Histologically, the changes in the muscles of the gizzard are hyaline necrosis and fibrosis.

Other Conditions Attributable to a Deficiency of Vitamin E

By feeding special diets to chicks, Dam and Glavind (*9*) produced a condition, which they called alimentary (nutritional) exudative diathesis, that could be cured by adding synthetic vitamin E (d,l alpha-tocopherol) to the diets. The condition was characterized by an accumulation of large quantities of transparent fluid in the subcutaneous tissues. The accumulations were found in various parts of the body but most frequently in the breast and abdomen. The fluid had the same composition as blood plasma and clotted readily. In addition to the accumulations of fluid, hyperemia (excess of blood), slight hemorrhage and accumulation of white blood corpuscles in connective tissues were observed.

Bird and Culton (*3*) have described a generalized edema which they produced in young chicks by feeding a diet of dried skim milk, dextrinized cornstarch, cod-liver oil and mineral salts. This diet is deficient in vitamin E and in other putritional factors, but Bird and, Culton were able to prevent the development of the edema by administering d,l alpha-tocopherol.

Hammond, at the Beltsville Research Center, Beltsville, Md., produced crazy-chick disease by feeding diets that contained 3 percent or more of cod-liver oil to day-old chicks. Mild cases were cured within a few days by administering synthetic vitamin E. This condition was essentially the same as the crazy-chick disease sometimes observed in commercial flocks and the brain lesions were like those found by Pappenheimer, Goettsch and Jungherr (*41*) in nutritional encephalomalacia.

Occurrence and Prevention of Vitamin E Deficiency

Crazy-chick disease, or nutritional encephalomalacia, occurs occasionally in commercial flocks that are fed typical feed mixtures for poultry. In such cases it has been often found that the feed mixture was prepared several months before it was used, strongly suggesting that the vitamin E originally in the feed was destroyed or inactivated before the feed was used.

Much can be done to avoid the destruction or inactivation of the vitamin E in feed mixtures by not using excessive quantities of cod-liver oil or other fats and oils and by feeding an mixtures within a short time after they are prepared.

Very few quantitative data are available on the vitamin E, content of feedstuffs and little is known about the quantitative requirements of poultry for vitamin E. It is known, however, that good sources of vitamin E include wheat-germ meal, alfalfa, alfalfa meal, alfalfa-leaf meal, wheat middlings, wheat shorts, wheat bran and an unground grains and seeds.

When nutritional encephalomalacia occurs in a flock, it can be checked and the individual cases that do not become acute can be cured, by adding to the diet 1 to 2 percent of corn oil, soyabean oil, peanut oil, wheat-germ oil, or cottonseed oil for a few weeks. Experience has shown that the addition to the diet of more than 2 percent of such oils is often much less effective than the addition of 1 percent.

Vitamin G Deficiency

The characteristic symptom of vitamin G deficiency in the chick is a condition referred to as curled-toe paralysis, but, according to Norris, Wilgus, Ringrose and others (*40*) and Stokstad and Manning (*48*), this condition does not occur if the diet is so extremely deficient in vitamin G that the chick dies. If a small quantity of vitamin G is added to an extremely deficient diet, the paralysis occurs, while if a sufficiently large quantity is added the paralysis is prevented. Three degrees of severity of curled-toe paralysis in chicks have been described by Stokstad and Manning (*48*). The first degree is characterized by a tendency to rest on the hocks and a slight curling of the toes, the second by marked weakness of the legs and a distinct curling of the toes of one or both feet and the third by toes that are completely curled inward or under and a weakened condition of the legs that compels the chicks to walk on their hocks.

Other symptoms of vitamin G deficiency in the chick are a marked decrease in the rate of growth or even complete failure to grow, diarrhea after 8 or 10 days and a high mortality rate after about 3 weeks. According to Lepkovsky and Jukes (*31*) the growth of the feathers appears not to be impaired. These workers have reported that, as a matter of fact, the main wing feathers appear to become disproportionately long.

The symptoms of vitamin G deficiency in the poult were found by Lepkovsky and Jukes (*31*) to be different from those in the chick. According to these workers, a dermatitis, or skin inflammation (Fig. 6), appears in young poults after about 8 days and the vent becomes encrusted, inflamed and excoriated, or stripped of skin. Growth slows up and ceases completely by about the seventeenth day and deaths begin to occur about the twenty-first day.

Findings After Death

According to Phillips and Engel (*42*) a deficiency of vitamin G in the diet of the chick produces specific changes in the main peripheral nerve trunks. In acute cases there are hypertrophy (increase in cell size) of the nerve trunks and a readily observable change in their appearance. Degenerative changes also appear in the myelin of the nerves. Phillips and Engel also found congestion and premature atrophy (wasting) of the lobes of the thymus. The kidney, thyroid and suprarenal glands, brain and brain stem appeared not to be affected.

Function of Vitamin G and Prevention of Deficiencies

It is know that vitamin G is an essential component of certain enzyme systems and that it has some functions in the oxidation processes of the cell. Just what happens when these enzyme systems fail is not definitely known, but the evidence available indicates that the growing chick requires vitamin G for the normal functioning and maintenance of the nervous system, particularly the main peripheral nerve trunks.

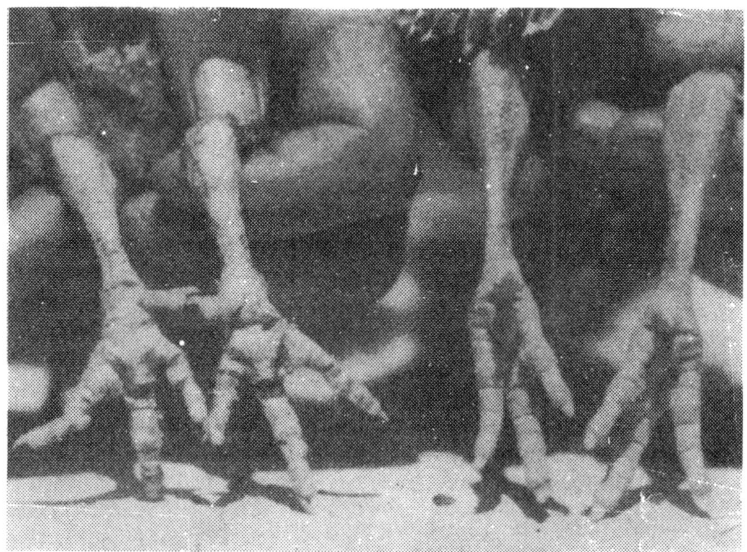

Fig. 6: Vitamin G deficiency in a turkey poult. Note the swelling, scaling, and fissuring in the feet of the poult at the left, produced by feeding a diet deficient in vitamin G. The poult whose normal feet are shown at the right received the same diet with the addition of a vitamin G concentrate made from whey. (Courtesy of Thomas H. Jukes, Division of Poultry Husbandry, California Agricultural Experiment Station, Davis, Calif).

Relatively few of the feedstuffs used for poultry contain enough vitamin G to meet the minimum requirement of the chick or poult during the first few weeks of life; hence if the ingredients of the diet of the young chick or poult are not selected so as to include one or more of the richer sources of vitamin G, the diet is likely to be deficient in this vitamin. In the case of chicks and poults that are closely confined this is especially true unless green feeds or other good sources of vitamin G, such as dried skim milk, dried buttermilk, and alfalfa-leaf meal are supplied.

The minimum vitamin G requirement of the growing chick and poult vanes with their age. During the first week it is about 1,300 micrograms per pound of feed for the chick and about 1,600 micrograms for the poult. The duckling's requirement is about the same as that of the chick. An adequate supply of vitamin G for the first 4 or 5 weeks for all three species is about 1,670 micrograms per pound of feed.

The vitamin G requirement of the adult chicken, turkey or duck is relatively low, but it increases somewhat with the onset of egg production. Chickens being kept for the eggs they produce; probably require only 600 to 800 micrograms of vitamin G per pound of feed, but the feed of breeding stock–chickens or turkeys–should contain about 1,250 micrograms per pound to maintain a high hatchability.

The approximate vitamin G contents of some of the richer sources of this vitamin used in feeding poultry are as follows:

	Micrograms per pound
Yeast, brewers', dried	16,000
Dried buttermilk (sweet cream)	12,000
Dried whey	10,000
Dried buttermilk	9,000
Dried skim milk	9,000
Alfalfa-leaf meal, dehydrated	8,000
Alfalfa-leaf meal	7,000
Alfalfa meal	5,000
Fish meal, whitefish	4,200
Fish meal, sardine	3,200
Meat scrap	3,000
Soybean meal	1,500

Vitamin K Deficiency

Apparently vitamin K is necessary for the formation of prothrombin, which in turn is necessary for the normal clotting of blood.

If very young chicks are fed a diet deficient in vitamin K, the time required for their blood to clot begins to increase after 5 to 10 days and becomes greatly increased after 7 to 12 days. After about a week on such a diet, hemorrhages often occur in any part of the body, spontaneously or as the result of an injury or bruise. The only external symptoms of vitamin K deficiency are the resulting accumulations of blood under the skin.

Chicks on a vitamin K deficient diet become anemic after a time as a result of the hemorrhages. Examination after death often reveals accumulations of blood in various parts of the body and there are invariably erosions of the gizzard lining (*1*).

The symptoms of vitamin K deficiency may be produced quite easily in young chicks m the labouratory, but they are seldom if ever observed when the chicks are raised in the usual manner. The age at which the vitamin K deficient diet is first fed influences the development of the resulting deficiency disease. The younger the chicks, the more susceptible they are; the deficient diet does not cause the disease after the chicks are a few weeks old. Hemorrhages may be produced within 12 to 20 days in adult chickens, however, by tying off the bile ducts, indicating that bile is necessary for the absorption of vitamin K.

Vitamin K has been found in such diverse materials as dried alfalfa, fish meal and rice bran that had been moistened and allowed to stand at room temperature for a few days, kale, tomatoes, hempseed meal and hog-liver fat. In corn, wheat, or rice there appears to be little or no vitamin K. In any case, it may be pointed out that in compounding practical diets for poultry it is not necessary to take special precautions to insure an adequate supply of vitamin K.

Pantothenic Acid Deficiency[6]

Symptoms

The symptoms of pantothenic acid deficiency is the chick, according to Ringrose, Norris and Heuser (*46*), are as follows: Growth is retarded and the feathers become ragged in appearance. Within 12 to14 days the margins of the eyelids become granulated and frequently a viscous exudate, which causes the eyelids to stick firmly together, is formed. Crusty scabs appear at the corners of the mouth (Fig. 7) and the skin on the bottoms of the feet often becomes thickened and cornified. At first there is no loss of down or feathers,

---

[6] The nutritional factor now called pantothenic acid has been referred to at various times as the chick antipellagra factor, the filtrate factor, the chick antidermatitis or antidermatosis factor, and the antidermatosis vitamin.

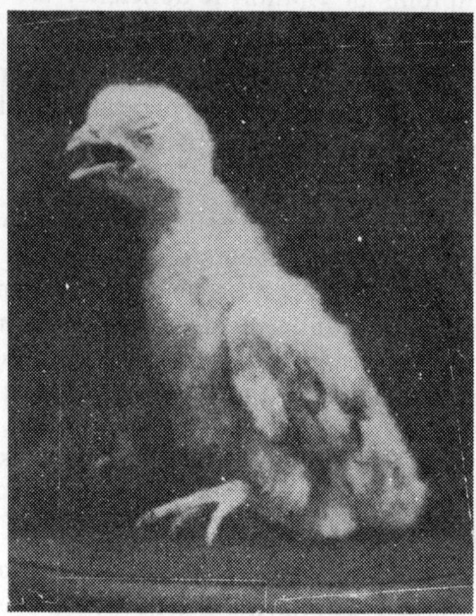

Fig. 7: Pantothenic-acid deficiency. Note the lesions at the corner of the mouth and on the eyelids, which are stuck together.

but after about 18 weeks complete loss of feathers in limited areas on the head and neck may occur.

The symptoms of pantothenic acid deficiency and egg-white injury (see the next section) are very similar, but according to Jukes[7] the two conditions may be distinguished from each other as follows: In egg-white injury the first symptom is a roughening of the skin below the lower mandible, whereas the dermatitis, or inflammation of the skin, observed in pantothenic acid deficiency appears first at the corners of the mouth and is seldom seen below the mandible. In egg-white injury the feet become involved at the same time as the mouth, whereas dermatitis of the feet is rarely seen in pantothenic acid deficiency and then only in the later stages–usually about 2 or 3 weeks after dermatitis has appeared at the corners of the mouth.

---

[7] Personal communication from T.H. Jukes, University of California, Davis, Calif.

The characteristic dermatitis produced in chicks by feeding diets deficient in pantothenic acid has not been found in adult chickens fed similar diets.

Findings After Death

Ringrose, Norris and Heuser (46) reported that on post mortem examination of the affected chicks a puslike substance was frequently observed in the mouth and an opaque, grayish-white exudate in the proventriculus. The entire intestinal tract was found to be almost entirely devoid of feed residues and the small intestine lacked normal tone and was atrophic (wasted). The liver frequently had an abnormal colour that varied from a faint yellow to a deep dirty yellow. The spleen appeared to be small and atrophic and the kidneys inflamed or hemorrhagic.

Phillips and Engel (43) found lesions in the spinal cord of chicks that had received a diet deficient in pantothenic acid. The lesions were characterized by a myelin degeneration (degeneration of the sheath) of the myelinated fibers. Such degenerating fibers were found in all segments of the spinal cord down to the lumbar region. Involution (degeneration) of the thymus and liver damage also were found.

The manner in which pantothenic acid functions in the chicken is not known, but the observations of Phillips and Engel show that it is necessary for the maintenance of a normal spinal cord in the growing chick.

Occurrence and Prevention of Pantothenic Acid Deficiency

Most of the feedstuffs ordinarily fed to poultry are fairly good sources of pantothenic acid, but diets composed largely or the cereal grains, wheat middlings and meat scrap or fish meal may contain less of this factor than is required by the growing chick. It should also be noted that the kiln-drying of corn tends to destroy much of the pantothenic acid originally present.

Cases of dermatosis (a general name for any skin disease) have been observed among growing chicks that were being raised under practical conditions and presumably were receiving an adequate diet. Undoubtedly there are causes of dermatosis other than a deficiency of pantothenic acid and it is possible that some them are nutritional, in nature. In the turkey, for example, a dermatosis may be produced by feeding a diet deficient in vitamin G.

The minimum pantothenic acid requirement of the chicken is set tentatively at about 5 milligrams per pound of feed. An adequate supply is about 6 milligrams per pound of feed, but apparently the diet of breeding stock should contain about 7 milligrams per pound of feed in order to insure good hatchability.

The approximate pantothenic acid contents of the richer sources of this vitamin, or vitamin like factor, that are used in feeding poultry are:

	Milligrams per pound
Yeast, brewers', dried	95
Cane molasses	6 to 38
Peanut meal	25
Dried whey	25
Dried buttermilk	19
Alfalfa-leaf meal, dehydrated	19
Dried skim milk	16
Alfalfa-leaf meal	13
Wheat bran	11
Rice bran	11
Soybean meal	6

Egg-White Injury

A condition in chicks that resembles pantothenic-acid-deficiency disease may be produced by feeding diets in which all or a rather large proportion of the animal protein is derived from egg white or from whole egg. It is called egg-white injury. Even as little as 5 percent of dried egg white or an equivalent quantity of liquid egg white in such diets produces a dermatitis at the corners of the mouth and on the bottoms of the feet.

Egg-white injury does not appear if 5 to 10 times as much egg yolk as egg white is also included in the diet. It may be prevented also by including relatively large quantities of dried skim milk, or about as much dried liver as egg white, or about half as much cooked pig kidney as egg white. If the egg white is cooked before it is dried, it does not produce the dermatitis.

The first symptoms of egg-white injury is the development of a dermatitis almost simultaneously at the corners of the mouth, below the lower mandible and on the bottoms of the feet. According to Jukes, however, roughening of the skin below the lower mandible is usually the first symptom to appear and is particularly noticeable where the skin joins the mandible. Later the eyes may be stuck shut and fissures appear in the skin on the bottoms of the feet. If the chicks survive long enough, the fissures become numerous and rather deep.

The precise cause of egg-white injury is not known, but it appears to result from a deficiency of biotin (vitamin H-one of the group of B vitamins). Apparently the egg white, if not denatured by cooking or otherwise, combines with and inactivates the biotin unless a rather large quantity is present in the diet.

Manganese and Choline Deficiencies[8]

Symptoms of Perosis

If young chicks are fed a diet deficient in manganese, symptoms of perosis will develop within 2 to 10 weeks, depending on the severity of the deficiency, the breed and strain of chicken, the composition of the diet and the age at which the diet is first led. If the deficient diet is fed from the first feeding, that is, when the chicks are 1 or 2 days old, the symptoms generally develop between the ages of 3 and 6 weeks, but if it is not fed until the chicks are 10 weeks old, the usual symptoms may not appear.

The first readily noticeable symptom is a tendency on the part of some of the chicks to rest for long periods in a squatting position. If the tibiotarsal joints (hocks) in these chicks are carefully examined, a slight puffiness may be observed. Within a few days the joints become slightly enlarged and frequently the skin covering them has a bluish-green cast. Apparently this is a critical stage, because in some cases, especially among the more resistant breeds or strains, the chicks frequently recover to such an extent that no readily noticeable permanent deformity results.

---

[8] This disease has been referred to at various times as hock disease, slipped tendon, and deforming leg weakness.

As the joints become further enlarged, they tend to become flattened and the metatarsi (shank bones) and tibiae exhibit a slight bending and also often undergo a rotational twisting. As the condition continues to develop, the bones become more and more bent until gross deformity results. Frequently the articular, or joint; cartilage at the lower end of the tibia slips from its normal position and this in turn causes the main tendons to slip from their condyies (the knucklelike ends of bones). Sometimes the curvature of a tibia is so great at its lower end that the tendons slip even though the articular cartilage has not been displaced. These changes may take place in either one or in both legs; when they take place in both legs the chicken is forced to walk on its hocks.

The symptoms of perosis in young poults and ducklings are similar to those observed in young chicks, but in the poult the next higher joint in the leg frequently becomes affected. Perosis has been found also in various wild birds, including pheasants, grouse, quail and sparrows.

Other Effects of a Deficiency of Manganese

If adult chickens are fed a diet deficient in manganese, no observable changes in their leg joints and bones occur, but the shells of their eggs tend to become thinner and less resistant to breakage. If the deficiency is sufficiently great, egg production is decreased and the eggs that are produced do not hatch well. The hatchability is reduced as a result of an increase in the embryonic mortality that occurs after the tenth day of incubation. According to Lyons and Insko (*33*) this embryonic mortality reaches its peak on the twentieth and twenty-first days of incubation and the embryos that die after the tenth day are chondrodystrophic and characterized by very short, thickened legs, short wings, "parrot beak," a globular contour of the head, protruding abdomen, and, in the most severe cases, retarded development of the down and poor growth.

If the deficiency of manganese in the diet of laying hens is marked but not extreme, a few of the eggs may hatch. The resulting chicks may have very short leg bones and in some cases the bones may be deformed as in chicks that develop perosis after hatching. Caskey and Norris (*8*) raised some of the short-legged chicks on diets that contained an adequate quantity of manganese and found that this condition of the legs persisted during a period much longer than that required for the attainment of maturity.

Chemical Findings and General Condition of the Bones in Perosis

The early work of Hall and King (*14*) indicated that chicks with slipped tendons had less bone phosphatase than normal chicks. Later Wiese, Johnson, Elvehjem and Hart (*52*) observed that both the blood and bone phosphatase and the ester phosphorus of the blood are decreased in manganese deficiency in the chick.

Although the majority of workers who have studied perosis in the chicken have reported that there is no material difference in the ash content of the leg bones in perotic and normal chicks, Caskey, Gallup and Norris (*7*) found that the leg bones of perotic chicks contained somewhat less ash than those of normal chicks.

Caskey, Gallup and Norris found also that a deficiency of manganese in the diet of chicks results in a significant thickening and shortening of the bones of the legs, wings and spinal column. In rickets, as in perosis, the leg bones may become thickened and shortened, but the shafts are poorly calcified and tough, whereas in perosis they are well calcified and relatively brittle. In osteoporosis the shafts are of normal length and much thinner than in rickets or perosis and are somewhat more springy than in perosis. In all three conditions the upper end of the tibia becomes enlarged, but it has a bulbous shape in rickets, a conical shape in perosis and an approximately normal shape in osteoporosis.

The Combined Action (Synergism) of Manganese and Choline

Soon after it was reported by Wilgus, Norris and Heuser (*54*) that manganese plays an important role in preventing perosis in growing chickens, seyeral workers observed that the addition of manganese to the diet was not in every case completely effective. In most instances no perosis occurred, but in a few instances 2 to 5 percent of the chicks developed relatively mild cases. Later it was found that the addition of manganese was less effective in preventing perosis in turkeys than in chickens.

Thus the matter stood until Jukes (*25, 26*) reported that choline, a widely distributed substance found in most animal and plant tissues, is effective in preventing perosis in both pouls and chicks if the diet contains manganese. Workers in several institutions soon confirmed Jukes' finding that the diet must contain adequate quantities of both manganese and choline if complete protection against perosis is to be obtained.

The manner in which manganese and choline function in the development of a normal skeleton is not yet known.

Occurrence and Prevention of Perosis

Perosis was seldom observed before the more intensive methods of raising poultry came into use. With development of out-of-season production of broilers it became a serious problem. In general, it occurred frequently whenever chickens and turkeys were raised without access to the soil. The reason is now apparent: only about 10 percent of the individual ingredients of mixed feeds for poultry contain enough manganese to furnish an adequate supply of this element and often these feedstuffs account for only 40 percent or less of the usual feed mixtures, but when poultry have access to the soil they ordinarily are able to obtain enough additional manganese to meet their requirement.

Corn and milk are extremely poor sources of manganese and diets composed largely of these two ingredients are likely to cause perosis, unless additional manganese is added. In the other hand, wheat bran, wheat middlings and rice bran are relatively rich sources and perosis is not likely to occur on diets that contain 20 percent or more of the first two or 10 percent of the third of these feedstuffs. In any case, it is good insurance against perosis to include a small quantity of manganese sulfate in the diet.

Most research workers in poultry nutrition agree that, for adequate protection against perosis, the diet of chickens should contain about 50 parts per million of manganese. Turkeys apparently require more manganese than chickens, but 50 to 60 parts per million will ordinarily meet their requirements, provided their diet also includes a sufficient quantity of choline.

In as much as most diets for poultry are likely to contain at least 20 parts per million of manganese, adequate protection against perosis generally will be obtained if about 30 parts per million are added. This quantity of manganese may be supplied easily through the use of a mixture of 100 parts, by weight, of common salt and 1.7 parts of pure anhydrous manganous sulfate, or about 2.2 parts of so-called technical grade anhydrous manganous sulfate. About 0.5 percent of this mixture, should be included in all-mash diets and 1 percent in mashes with which an approximately equal quantity of grain is to be fed.

Nearly all the feedstuffs commonly used in feeding poultry contain, some choline, so that typical diets for poultry are not likely to be deficient in this substance. One of the better sources of choline among feedstuffs is Soybean meal and for this reason, the, inclusion of 5 to 10 percent of this feedstuff in diets for poultry, especially for turkeys, will tend to insure against a deficiency of choline.

Iron and Copper Deficiencies and Anemia

Anemia rarely if ever occurs among chickens on practical diets, but it has been demonstrated (*10, 16*) that it can be produced in young chicks by feeding a diet extremely deficient in iron or Copper or both. The workers cited produced anemia in young chicks by feeding a diet of cow's milk, polished rice, calcium carbonate and salt and a similar diet in which the rice was replaced by corn.

When the rice-containing diet was fed, the hemoglobin content of the blood fell from 8 grams per 100 cubic centimeters to 4 grams per 100 cubic centimeters within 12 to 15 days. The anemia was prevented by adding a small quantity of a soluble salt of iron to the diet. However, if the rice was first treated to remove the small quantity of copper it contained, it was necessary to add salts of both iron and copper to obtain normal hemoglobin formation.

When the corn-containing diet was fed, anemia developed during the early growing period but gradually disappeared as the chicks became older. As in the case of the rice-containing diet, the addition of iron prevented the occurrence of anemia.

As was found by Hogan and Parrott (22), anemia can also be produced in young chicks by feeding special, simplified diets that presumably have an adequate content of iron and copper. In such instances the anemia is the result of a deficiency of some as yet unknown nutritional factor.

Although anemia of nutritional origin occurs extremely rarely in chickens, it has been observed in developing embryos in eggs from hens that had received more or less typical diets for poultry. Anemic embryos are encountered most frequently in the fall and winter, when the parent stock does not receive much sunshine. The exact cause of this anemia in embryos is not known, but probably the cause is a deficiency of iron or copper or both. At least there is evidence that if chickens do not receive sunshine or do not have some cod-liver oil in their diet, the transfer of iron and copper to their eggs is appreciably reduced.

The available evidence on the subject indicates that under ordinary, practical conditions it is unnecessary to add compounds of iron and copper to the diets of poultry to prevent anemia. As a matter of fact, the addition of large quantities of iron compounds may produce rickets by making the phosphorus unavailable.

Iodine Deficiency and Goiter

Only a few cases of goiter, or enlarged thyroid (Fig. 8), in chickens have been observed and reported in this country, but Welch (*51*) has stated that it is very common in Montana and Kernkamp (*28*) has reported two cases in Minnesota Goiter in the chicken probably is more common in certain sections of this country than is generally realized, Undoubtedly the reason that only a few cases have been

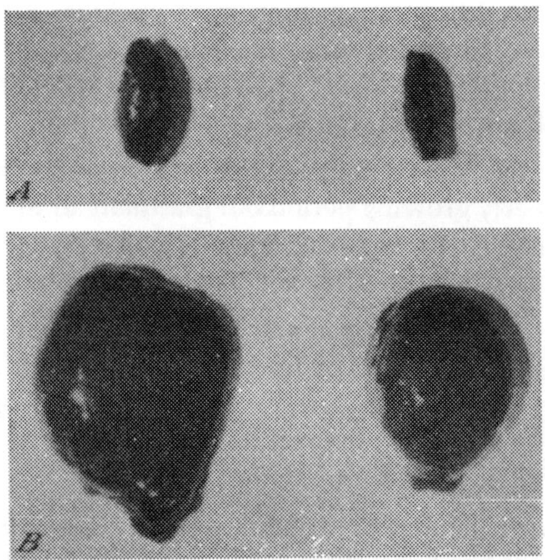

Fig. 8: *A*: normal, and *B*: enlarged thyroid glands of chickens. The enlarged thyroid was removed from a chicken that had been fed a diet deficient in iodine. (Courtesy of H.S. Wilgus, Colorado Agricultural Experimental Station, For Collins, Colo).

reported is that the enlarged thyroids are concealed by the feathers and are not readily detected, Moreover, goiter does not appear to affect the health of chickens seriously or to be a cause of heavy mortality.

Goiter has been produced experimentally in chickens by Gassner and Wilgus (*13*). They fed diets of extremely low iodine content (25 parts per billion) to laying hens and found enlarged thyroid glands in the chicks that hatched from their eggs. Wilgus and associates (*53*) were able to produce goiter in young growing chicks by feeding them a simplified diet of low iodine content in which the sole protein supplement was soybeans. However, when they added sufficient iodine to this diet the thyroid glands were normal in size and structure.

Such experiments have provide definite evidence that the chicken requires a small quantity of iodine, but neither the minimum nor the optimum amount is known. Mitchell and McClure (*37*) estimated that the daily iodine requirement of a 5-pound chicken is 4.5 to 9 micrograms (a microgram is one-millionth of a gram, or slightly less than one twenty-eight millionth of an ounce).

Most American workers who have studied the effect of adding small quantities of iodine to the diet of chickens have reported that no beneficial results were obtained, which suggests that typical diets for poultry are not likely to be deficient in iodine. Nevertheless, the use of so-called iodized salt in diets for poultry–especially in sections of the country where goiter is encountered in other farm, animals–may be a worth-while means of insuring against a possible deficiency of iodine.

Gizzard Erosion

Several different kinds of gizzard erosion are found in poultry and the meager evidence now available suggests that they are the result of different causes or combinations of causes. The kind most frequently encountered is preceded by hemorrhages from the glandular layer of the gizzard, which originate from the capillaries in the submucosa. A second kind, which is less common, is characterized by a softening and a pronounced thickening of the lining of the gizzard. In a third kind, which is of still less frequent occurrence and has been observed chiefly in turkeys, the lining softens and separates completely from the glandular layer. The last kind of erosion is distinctly different from the first but resembles the second in that there is a softening of the lining.

Little or nothing is known about the development of the second and third kinds of gizzard erosion, but the histological studies of Lansing, Miller and Titus (*30*) have yielded some information regarding the development of the first kind, which is discussed in the following paragraphs.

According to these authors the erosions are formed in the following way:

At one or more places in the glandular layer of the gizzard there is a seepage of blood into the secretion from which the lining is formed, and the lining is thus weakened in these places and loses some of its coherence. Reddishbrown stains in the lining varying in size from a mere speck to several square centimeters are evidence of such seepage. If the passage of blood into the secretion stops at this stage, the subsequent secretion yields a normal layer of lining under the affected area. After a short time threadlike, shallow fissures appear on the attrition surface of the lining in such places.

Sometimes the initial seepage of blood is followed by a pronounced hemorrhage and blood clots form between the weakened lining and the glandular layer. If the seepage continues for some time before the hemorrhage occurs, a fairly thick but deeply stained lining may be found over the blood clot; but if the hemorrhage follows promptly after the initial seepage, only a thin lining or no lining at all is found over the site of the hemorrhage. In either case, the affected portion of the lining now lacks the backing or support of the glandular layer and soon cracks or sloughs off. The final result is the formation of deeply fissured areas, holes in the lining, or both.

Apparently, when the hemorrhages are large the secreting activity of the glands is markedly reduced or even stopped. In any case, new lining is not formed and large eroded areas appear.

If at any stage in the development of gizzard erosions a suitable diet is fed, the hemorrhages stop, and, after 2 or 3 weeks a lining of normal appearance may be formed.

Gizzard erosion has been found in all sections of the country and presumably in all breeds of chickens. Its incidence is greatest in very young chicks and decreases with increasing age.

Apparently gizzard erosion has no appreciable effect on the rate of growth or the health of chickens. In any case, its occurrence in very young chicks is not a cause for concern. If it is found in chicks older than 4 weeks, however, the diet fed is probably not entirely satisfactory.

Various feedstuffs and other materials have been reported to be of value in clearing up gizzard erosion. Among those reputed to be of special value are dried ox bile, cholic acid, kale, hempseed meal, alfalfa products, wheat bran, wheat middlings, oats, soybean meal, pig liver and kidney, lung tissue, cartilage and chondroitin. Of these materials the most effective are dried ox bile and cholic acid.

The diverse nature of the materials just mentioned strongly suggests that gizzard erosion may result from a deficiency of more than one nutritional factor and that the deficiency may be single or multiple. This suggestion is strengthened by the fact that although dried ox bile has been very effective in the experiments of all workers who have tested it, some workers have failed to get a response from cartilage and chondroitin and others have obtained very little if any response from alfalfa.

Feather Picking and Cannibalism

Cannibalism is a term used by some poultrymen in referring to the habit sometimes developed by chickens, turkeys, other poultry and game birds of picking one another's feathers, toes, beaks, heads, combs, backs, vents and other parts of the body. Some poultrymen, however, restrict the use of this term to cases in which blood is drawn. In as much as there are instances in which only the feathers are picked, or pulled, it seems desirable to make a distinction between feather picking and cannibalism.

Often the only result of feather picking is that some of the birds lose many of their feathers, but cannibalism nearly always leads to heavy losses through death. In flocks of pullets just starting to lay, cannibalism generally follows a case of prolapsus of the oviduct; in such cases a number of birds may become disemboweled and rather heavy losses may result. Cannibalism among chicks often appears first in the form of toe picking, back picking, or wing picking; once established, it spreads rapidly through the flock.

Although there is evidence that feather picking and cannibalism are the result, in part, of unsatisfactory diets, there are often other contributing causes, such as overcrowding and overheating–especially in the case of chicks in battery brooders. The exact nature of the nutritional deficiency or deficiencies involved is not known, but it has been found that feather picking and cannibalism are less likely to occur if the diet contains about 20 percent of barley or oats or about 30 percent of bran and middlings.

Carver (*6*) has reported that feather picking and cannibalism may be controlled by using ruby-coloured lights in place of ordinary lights in battery brooders and brooder houses. Miller and Hearse (*35*) have reported that if oats are fed as the sole grain in diets for growing and laying pullets, cannibalism is significantly reduced. They found that the effective part of the oats was the hulls. Their findings and those of other workers indicate that feather picking and cannibalism are likely to appear if diets of very low crude-fiber content are fed.

One of the most effective methods of stopping feather picking and cannibalism is to increase the salt content of the diet for 2 or 3 days. If an all-mash diet is being fed, add 2 percent of salt, but if both mash and grain are being fed, add 4 percent of salt to the mash. Usually the feather picking or cannibalism stops within a few hours, but in some cases 2 or 3 days may be required. It should be noted that the salt treatment is recommended as a curative rather than a preventive measure; that is, it is not recommended that more than 0.5 to 0.7 percent of added salt be included regularly in all-mash diets or that more than 1 to 1.2 percent be included in mashes with which grain is fed.

Among poultrymen there is a fairly common belief that salt is poisonous to poultry and for that reason they may be somewhat reluctant to use the salt treatment. Salt is poisonous to an animals if consumed in large single doses; Mitchell, Card and Carman (*36*) have reported, however, that a daily intake of 6 to 8 grams (about 0.2 to 0.3 ounce) of salt mixed in the feed appears to have no harmful effect on chickens 9 weeks or more of age. They found that the minimum lethal dose for chickens weighing 3 to 5 pounds is equivalent to about 0.4 percent of their live weight. When the salt treatment is used, the largest quantity of salt likely to be consumed by an adult bird in a day is about 5 grams; that likely to be consumed by a growing bird is usually much less. It is thus clear that there is no danger of so-called salt poisoning when the salt treatment is used.

If the salt treatment is not effective after 2 or 3 days, it may be necessary to trim or sear back to the quick the upper mandible of the beaks of all the birds. The trimming may be done with a sharp knife, the searing with a hot soldering iron. When carefully done, the operation is painless. Ordinarily, only about three-sixteenths of an inch of the tip of the beak is removed; the proper amount can be judged readily by the appearance of the beak substance.

Fluorine Poisoning

Although the tolerance of chickens for fluorine is greater than that of cattle le and swine, the continued ingestion of diets containing appreciable quantities may depress the rate of growth and the egg production. Fluorine is distributed almost universally in plants and feedstuffs, as well as in animal tissues, but the quantity present is usually very small. Danger of fluorine toxicosis, or poisoning, in chickens exists only when the drinking water contains about 2 parts or million or more of fluorine or when rock phosphate or phosphatic limestone is included in the diet. Apparently the only observable effects of fluorine toxicosis are those it has on growth and egg production.

Most of the available information about the effects of fluorine on chickens has been obtained from experiments conducted at the Wisconsin and Ohio experiment stations.

Experiments by Halpin and Lamb (*15*) at the Wisconsin station; showed that the inclusion in the diet of chicks of 1 percent of rock phosphate that contained about 3.5 percent of fluorine had no harmful effect, but the inclusion of 2 percent depressed the growth to some extent and the inclusion of 3 percent had a more marked effect. Only the highest of the three levels of rock phosphate in the diet of pullets tended to decrease egg production.

At the Ohio experiment station the studies of Kick, Bethke and Record (*29*) showed that chicks can tolerate a larger quantity of fiuorine in the form of calcium fluoride than in the form of sodium fluoride; the fluorine in rock phosphate also was more toxic than that in the calcium fluoride. They concluded that when the diet of chicks contains more than 0.036 percent of fluorine, from either sodium fluoride or rock phosphate, feed consumption and growth are decreased in proportion to the fluorine content of the diet. However, according to Hauck, Steenbock, Lowe and Halpin (*17*) diets that contain as much as 0.068 percent of fluorine in the form of sodium fluoride may be fed to chicks without affecting their growth. In any case it is apparently not advisable to include rock phosphate or phosphatic limestone in diets for poultry.

Selenium Poisoning

Practically all our knowledge of selenium toxicosis in poultry has resulted from studies conducted at the South Dakota Agricultural Experiment Station. It should be pointed out, however, that South Dakota is not the only State in which selenium toxicosis may be encountered. According to Moxon (*38*) selenium has been found in the soils and vegetation of at least 11 of the States in the Great Plains and the Rocky Mountains and it is probably present in the soils of other States in these regions.

Poley, Moxon and Franke (*45*) found that if laying chickens were fed diets that contained grain in which the selenium content was about 15 parts per million, feed consumption decreased appreciably, the chickens lost weight and after about a week none of their eggs would hatch. Tully and Franke (*49*) observed that it chicks were fed a diet that contained 65 percent of the toxic grain their growth was definitely inhibited and their feathers became ruffled. The egg production of the pullets raised on such diets was both delayed and reduced.

In later studies Poley and Moxon (*44*) found that if the diet of laying chickens contained only 2½ parts per million of selenium, hatchability was not appreciably affected; if the diet contained about 5 parts per million of selenium, however, the hatchability was reduced somewhat; and if it contained 10 parts per million the hatchability soon decreased to zero. The decrease in hatchability was attributed to abnormal development of the embryos, most of which died before the twenty-first day of incubation. The most prominent deformity among the abnormal embryos was the lack of a full-sized upper beak. Other abnormalities were the absence of eyes, feet and wings, wiry down and edema of the head and neck.

Other Diseases of Nutritional Chicken

Several poultry-nutrition workers, while studying the effects of feeding simplified diets, have encountered various abnormal conditions in poultry that apparently could not have been caused by a deficiency of any known nutritional factor. However, the very fact that simplified diets were being fed suggests that the abnormal conditions were of nutritional origin. One such condition, the anemia described by Hogan and Parrott (22), has been mentioned in a preceding section; others are enteritis (intestinal inflammation), paralysis, arthritis, dermatosis and fatty liver; undoubtedly there are still others.

Certain abnormal conditions, such as enteritis, dermatosis and fatty liver have been observed even when supposedly adequate diets were being fed. As more is learned about the nutritional requirements of poultry and the nutritive properties of feedstuffs, it is probable that the causes of these abnormal conditions will be found.

Enteritis

Enteritis or inflammation of the intestine-chiefly the small intestine-is frequently observed in chickens that are being raised without access to the soil and green growing plants. On autopsy, the intestine is often found to be filled with bits of shavings, straw, or other material that had been used as litter; sometimes large quantities of grit are also found. A somewhat similar but more severe condition, called ulcerative enteritis, causes heavy losses among quail, pheasants, grouse and wild turkeys that are being raised in captivity.

Attempts to demonstrate that such conditions are caused by a microorganism or other causative agent have failed. It has been suggested that in game birds the immediate cause is a diet of high fiber content, but enteritis is frequently encountered among both chickens and quail fed diets of comparatively low fiber content.

Paralysis

As has been pointed out in preceding sections, a deficiency of vitamin E in the diet of the young growing chicken produces lesions in the brain, of pantothenic acid in the spinal cord, of vitamin G in the main peripheral nerve trunks, of vitamin A in the central and peripheral nervous systems. Moreover, a dietary deficiency of vitamin B_1 produces a toxicosis, or poisoning, of the nervous system. Accordingly, a deficiency of one or more of these vitamins may pro. duce paralysis or a similar condition.

Paralysis of nutritional origin has been observed, however, when adequate quantities of all five of the vitamins just mentioned were supplied. For example, Jukes and Babcock (*27*) have described a paralysis that could be prevented by supplementing the diet with alfalfa meal or a water extract of alfalfa and Bird and Oleson (*4*) have described a condition, in which there is in co-ordination of the leg muscles, which they attribute to a deficiency of vitamin B_4. According to Hegsted, Oleson, Elvehjem and Hart (*19*) the latter condition is not prevented by alfalfa or vitamin E but is prevented by relatively large quantities of dried brain, cartilage, wheat middlings, yellow corn, or wheat.

Arthritis

In 1935 Van der Boom, Branion and Graham (*50*) described a deformity of the legs of chickens that resulted from feeding simplified diets that contained highly purified casein. They tentatively called the condition arthritis. Later Branion and his associates (*5*) concluded that this condition is probably the result of a deficiency of one or more inorganic elements. Still later other workers (*19*) suggested that the "paralysis" (see the preceding discussion of paralysis) that they had encountered in the chicken might be the same as the "arthritis" reported by Van der Hoorn, Branion and Graham (*50*).

According to the latter authors, the first symptom of this arthritis appeared, when the chicks were about 3 weeks old. At first the chicks were merely less active than usual, but within a few days they showed very little inclination to walk and when they did walk their gait was decidedly stilted and there was practically no flexion of the tibiotarsal (hock) joints. At this stage the capsule of the joint was swollen and somewhat congested and there was a slight excess of fluid in the cavity. Gradually the symptoms became more pronounced until the chicks refused to walk. Often the leg bones became deformed as in perosis, but the investigators concluded that their "arthritis" was not perosis.

Dermatosis

From time to time a dermatosis similar to that produced by a deficiency of pantothenic acid or to that which results from the feeding of egg white is observed among growing chickens that are receiving supposedly adequate diets. This condition often disappears if a complete change of diet is made, but it is not cured by adding rich sources of pantothenic acid to the original diet.

Hegsted and associates (*18*) have reported such a condition occurring among chicks that were led a purifier diet in which there was an adequate supply of pantothenic acid. In many respects the symptoms were the same as those of egg-white injury and complete cures were obtained by injecting a potent preparation of vitamin H (biotin). Hegsted and associates concluded that it is possible that all proteins have the effect of egg white to some extent but that the effect would be evidence only when purified diets low in the protective factor are fed.

Fatty Liver

When growing chickens are fed certain simplified diets, their livers often have an abnormal yellow colour and show evidence of fatty degeneration. Lepkovsky, Taylor, Jukes and Almquist (*32*) have reported that a deficiency of vitamin G (riboflavin) causes fatty liver in chicks and Engel and Phillips (*12*) have reported that when vitamin B_1 is administered to chicks that have been on a diet deficient in this vitamin a similar condition develops. However, Hegsted, Oleson, Elvehjem and Hart (*19*) have described a fatty degeneration of the liver that could not be attributed to either of the causes just mentioned.

The available evidence indicates that fatty liver in chickens may be the result of a number of causes and not a single, specific nutritional deficiency. When fatty liver is found, however, it may be concluded that the diet is unsatisfactory, as a result either of one or more deficiencies or of an imbalance of certain nutritional factors.

Effect of Nutritional Deficiencies on Growth and Reproduction

Although an animal's capacity to grow is an inherited character, the growth it makes depends on its nutrition. The dependence of growth on nutrition is so great that when an adequate diet is fed the relationship between live weight and feed consumption may be expressed with a high degree of accuracy by a mathematical equation. When an inadequate diet is fed, the animal's growth is usually retarded and irregular. Often a retardation of growth is the first indication that the diet is deficient.

A fairly large number of nutritive factors are required for normal growth. Among those that play especially prominent roles in maintaining growth in poultry are vitamins A, B_1, B_6, D and G (Fig. 9), pantothenic acid, glucuronic acid, choline, several of the amino acids and many of the inorganic elements. Apparently, there are other vitamins or vitaminlike factors that affect growth, but very little is yet known about them.

Obviously, a retardation of growth merely indicates that the diet is inadequate. Only when other symptoms appear, or when information about the diet that is being fed is fairly complete, is it possible to identify the deficiency. The symptoms of a number of nutritional deficiencies have already been described.

Egg production sometimes continues even though a deficient diet is fed. Likewise the fertility of the eggs appears not to be greatly, affected by dietary deficiencies unless they are acute and prolonged enough to affect the health of the birds, especially that of the males.

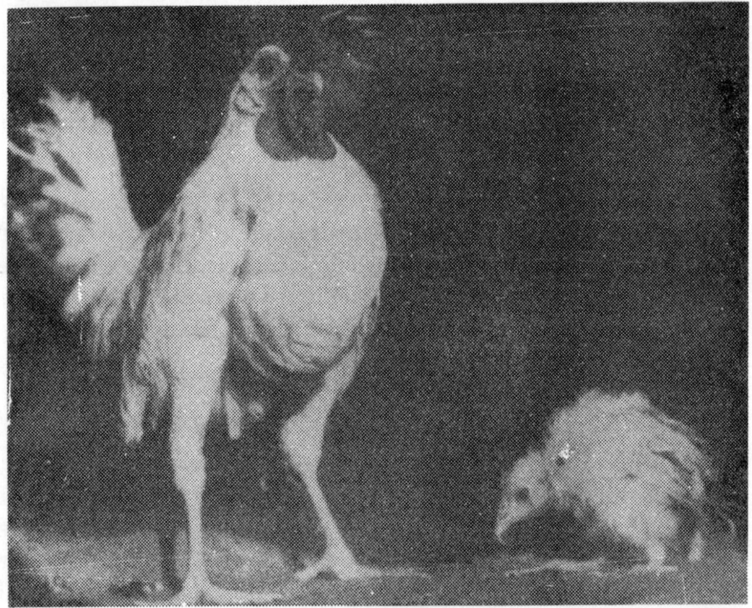

Fig. 9: Many nutritional deficiencies retard growth. Both these chickens are 114 days old. The one at the left received an ordinary mixed diet; the one at the right received a diet deficient in vitamin G. (Courtesy of Thomas H. Jukes, Division of Poultry Husbandry, California Agricultural Experiment Station, Davis, Calif.).

The hatchability of the eggs is readily decreased by a number of dietary deficiencies. However, as a matter of fact, the first and frequently the only indication that the diet of adult birds is deficient in one or more nutritive factors is a low hatchability of the eggs.

Among the nutritional factors known to be required for the production of hatchable eggs are vitamins A, D, E and G, pantothenic acid, protein of good quality, calcium and manganese. To this list may be added the "alcohol-precipitate factor" of Schumacher and Heusel (47). Undoubtedly, other factors are required and as more work is done they will be discovered and described.

Nutritional deficiencies are not the only causes of poor hatchability. As was mentioned in the discussion of selenium poisoning, if the diet of the dams contains as much as 10 parts per million of selenium none of their eggs will hatch. Moreover, the inclusion of excessively large quantities of calcium or phosphorus in the diet also decreases hatchability.

Just how a deficiency of vitamin A in the diet of the dams affects the development of the embryos in their eggs is not known, but the ultimate effect–a decreased hatchability–may be easily demonstrated.

When the diet of the dams is deficient in vitamin D, the embryos in their eggs are unable to obtain enough calcium and phosphorus and the embryonic mortality reaches a peak on the eighteenth or nineteenth day of incubation. An excessive intake of vitamin D (5 or 6 times the normal requirement) also decreases the hatchability of the eggs.

A vitamin E deficiency in the diet of the dams is manifested by a marked increase in the embryonic death rate between the third and fifth days of incubation.

When there is a deficiency of vitamin G or of protein of good quality, a marked increase in the so-called second-week embryonic mortality occurs.

A deficiency of pantothenic acid in the diet reduces the hatchability of the eggs, but no characteristic peak of embryonic mortality has been reported.

A deficiency of calcium in the diet seems to have an effect similar to that of a deficiency of vitamin D. An excess of either calcium or phosphorus causes an increase in embryonic mortality during the last 3 days of the incubation period.

The effect on the embryos of feeding diets deficient in manganese to chickens has been previously discussed.

Literature Cited

(1) ALMQUIST, H.J. and STOKSTAD, E.L.R. (1935). HEMORRHAGIC CHICK DISEASE OF DIETARY ORIGIN. Jour. Biol. Chem. 111: 105-113.

(2) BARGER, EDGAR HUGH and CARD, LESLIE ELLSWORTH (1938). DISEASES AND PARASITES OF POULTRY. Ed. 2, 386 pp., illus. Philadelphia.

(3) BIRD, H.R. and CULTON, THOS, G. (1940). GENERALIZED EDEMA IN CHICKS PREVENTED BY D, L-ALPHA TOCOPHEROL. Soc. Expt. Biol. and Med. Proc. 44(2): 543-547, illus.

(4) _____and OLESON, J.J. (1938). VITAMIN A DEFICIENCY IN CHICKS FFD PURIFIED RATIONS CONTAINING COD LIVER OIL. Soc. Expt. Biol. and Med. Proc. 38: 870-871.

(5) BRANION, H.D., MARTIN, R.L., ROBERTSON, E.B. and others (1938). THE VARIATION IN THE NUTRITIVE VALUE OF CASEIN. Poultry Sci. 17: 301-316.

(6) CARVER, J.S. (1931). THE CONTROL OF CANNIBALISM IN BATTERY BROODERS AND FATTENING BATTERIES. Poultry Sci. 10: 275-277.

(7) CASKEY, C.D., GALLUP, W.D. and NORRIS, L.C. (1939). THE NEED FOR MANGANESE IN THE BONE DEVELOPMENT OF THE CHICK. Jour. Nutr. 17: 407-417, illus.

(8) _____and NOBRIS, L.C. ((1940). MICROMELIA IN ADULT FOWL CAUSED BY MANGANESE DEFICIENCY DURING EMBRYONIC DEVELOPMENT. Soc. Expt. Biol. and Med. Proc. 44; 332-335, illus.

(9) DAM, HENRIK and GLAVIND, JOHANNES (1940). VITAMIN E AND KAPILLARPERMEABILITAT. Naturwissenschaften 28: 207.

(10) ELVEHJEM, C.A. and HART, E.B. (1929). THE RELATION OF IRON AND COPPER TO HAEMOGLOBIN SYNTHESIS IN THE CHICK. Jour. Biol. Chem. 84: 131-141.

(11) ENGEL, R.W. and PHILLIPS, P.H. (1938). THE LACK OF NERVE DEGENERATION IN UNCOMPLICATED VITAMIN B_1 DEFOCIENCY IN THE CHICK AND THE RAT. Jour. Nutr. 16: 585-596.

(12) _____and PHILLIPS, P.H. (1939). FATTY LIVERS AS A RESULT OF THIAMIN ADMINISTRATION IN VITAMIN B_1 DEFICIENCY OF THE RAT AND THE CHICK. Jour. Nutr. 18(4): 329- 338, illus.

(13) GASSNER, F.X., and WILGUS, H.S. (1940). CONGENITAL GOITER IN CHICKS. (Abstract of paper) Poutry Sci. 19: 349.

(14) HALL, G.E. and KING, EARL J. (1931). CALCIUM AND PHOSPHORUS METABOLISM IN THE CHICKEN. II. "RANGE PARALYSIS." Poultry Sci. 10: 259-268, illus.

(15) HALPIN, J.G. and LAMB, ALVIN R. (1932). THE EFFECT OF GROUND PHOSPHATE ROCK FED AT VARIOUS LEVELS ON THE GROWTH OF CHICKS AND ON EGG PRODUCTION. Poultry Sci. 11: 5-13.

(16) HART, E.B., ELVEHJEM, C.A. KEMMERER, A.R. and HALPIN, J.G. (1930). DOES THE PRACTICAL CHICK RATION NEED IRON AND COPPER ADDITIONS TO INSURE NORMAL HEMOGLOBIN BUILDING? Poultry Sci. 9: 92-101.

(17) HAUCK, HAZEL M., STEENBOOK, H., LOWE, JAMES T. and HALPIN, J.G. (1933). EFFECT OF FLUORINE ON GROWTH, CALCIFICATION AND PARATHYRPODS IN THE CHICKEN. Poultry Sci. 12: 242-249, illus.

(18) HEGSTED, D. MARK, OLESON, J.J., MILLS, R.C. and others (1940). STUDIES ON A DERMATITIS IN CHICKS DISTINCT FROM PANTOTHENIC ACID DEFICIENCY. Jour. Nutr. 20: 599-606, illus.

(19) _____OLESON, J.J., ELVEHJEM, C.A. and HART, E.B. (1940). THE ESSENTIAL NATURE OF A NEW GROWTH FACTOR AND VITAMIN B_6 FOR CHICKS. Poultry Sci. 19: 167-176.

(20) HEYWANG, BURT W. and MORGAN, RUDOLPH B. (1937). OBSERVATIONS ON SOME SYMPTOMS OF VITAMIN A DEFICIENCY IN CHICKS. Poultry Sci. 16: 388-392, illus.

(21) HINSHAW, W.R. and LLOYD, W.E. (1934). VITAMIN-A DEFIENCY IN TURKEYS, Hilgardia 8: 281-304, illus.

(22) HOGAN, ALBERT G. and PARROTT, ERNEST M. (1940). ANEMIA IN CHICKS CAUSED BY A VITAMIN DEFICIENCY. Jour. Biol. Chem. 132: 507-517, illus.

(23) JUKES, THOMAS H. (1939). VITAMIN B_6 DEFICIENCY IN CHICKS. Soc. Expt. Biol. and Med. Proc. 42: 180-182., illus.

(24) _____(1940). EFFECT OF YEAST EXTRACT AND OTHER SUPPLEMENTS ON THE GROWTH OF CRICKS FED SIMPLIFIED DIETS. Jour. Biol. Chem. 133: 631-632.

(25) _____(1940). PREVENTION OF PEROSIS BY CHOLINE. Jour. Biol. Chem. 134: 789-790.

(26) _____(1940). EFFECT OF CHOLINE AND OTHER SUPPLEMENTS ON PEROSIS. Jour. Nutr. 20: 445-458, illus.

(27) _____and BABOOCK, SIDNEY H., JR. (1938). EXPERIMENTS WITH A FACTOR PROMOTING GROWTH AND PREVENTING PARALYSIS IN CHICKS ON A SIMPLIFIED DIET. Jour. Biol. Chem. 125: 169-181, illus.

(28) KERNKAMP, H.C.H. (1925). GOITER IN POULTRY. Amer. Vet. Med. Assoc. Jour. 67: 223-228, illus.

(29) KICK, C.H., BETHKE, R.M., RECORD, P.R. (1933). EFFECT OF FLUORINE ON THE NUTRITION OF THE CHICK, Poultry Sci. 12: 382-387.

(30) LANSING, ALBERT., MILLER, DAVID and TITUS, HARRY W. (1939). THE FORMATION OF EROSIONS OF THE GIZZARD LINING IN THE YOUNG CHICK. Poultry Sci. 18: 475-480, illus.

(31) LEPKOVSKY, SAMUEL and JUKES, THOMAS H. (1936). THE RERPONSE OF RATS; CHICKS AND POULTS TO CRYSTALLINE VITAMIN G (FLAVIN). Jour. Nutr. 12: 515-526, illus.

(32) _____TAYLOR, L.W., JUKES, T.H. and ALMQUIST, H.J. (1938). THE EFFECT OF RIBOFLAVIN AND THE FILTRATE FACTOR ON EGG PRODUCTION AND HATCHABILITY. Hilgardia 11: 559-591, illus.

(33) LYONS, MALCOLM and INSKO, W.M., JR. (1937). CHONDRODYSTROPHY IN THE CHICK EMBRYO PRODUCED BY MANGANESE DEFICIENCY IN THE DIET OF THE HEN. Ky. Agr. Expi. Sta. Bul. 371: 61-75, illus.

(34) McGOWAN, JOHN POOL and EMSILIE, ARTHUR RAYMOND GORDON (1934). RICKETS IN CHICKENS, WITH SPECIAL REFERENCE TO ITS NATURE AND PATHOOENESIS. Biochem. Jour. 28: [1500]-1512, illus.

(35) MILLER, M. WAYNE and BEARSE, GORDON E. (1937). THE CANNIBALISM PREVENTING PROPERTIES OF OATS. Poultry Sci. 16: 314-321.

(36) MITCHELL, H.H.,·CARD, L.E. and CARMAN, G.G., (1926). THE TOXICITY OF SALT FOR CHICKENS. Ill. Agr. Expt. Sta. Bul. 279: 133-156, illus.

(37) _____and McCLURE, F.J. (1937). MINERAL NUTRITION OF FARM ANIMALS. Natl. Res. Council Bul. 99, 135 pp.

(38) MOXON, ALVIN L. (1937). ALKALI DISEASE OR SELENIUM POISONING. S. Dak. Agr. Expt. Sta. BuL. 311, 91 pp., illus.

(39) NITZESCU, I.I. and IOANID, V. (1940). LA GLYCEMIE CHEZ LES POULES EN AVITAMINOSE Dl. SOC. de Biol. [Paris] Compt. Rend. 133; 400-491, illus.

(40) NORRIS, L.C., WILGUS, B.S., JR., RINGROSE, A.T. and others (1936). THE VITAMIN-G REQUIREMENT OF POULTRY. N.Y. (Cornell) Agr. Expt. Sta. Bul. 660, 20 pp., illus.

(41) PAPPENHEIMER, ALWIN M., GOETTSCH, MARIANNE and JUNGHERR, ERWIN (1939). NUTRITIONAL ENCEPHALOMALACIA IN CHICKS AND CERTAIN RELATED DISORDERS OF DOMESTIC BIRDS. Conn. (Storrs) Expt. Sta. Bul. 229, 121 pp:, illus.

(42) PHILLIPS, PAUL B. and ENGEL, R.W. (1938). THE HISTOPATHOLOGY OF NEUROMALACIA AND "CURLED TOE" PARALYSIS IN THE CHICK FED LOW RIBOFLAVIN DIETS. Jour. Nutr. 16: 451-463, illus.

(43) _____and ENGEL, R.W. (1939). SOME HISTOPATHOLOGIC OBSERVATIONS ON CHICKS DEFICIENT IN THE CHICK ANTIDERMATITIS FACTOR OR PANTOTHENIC ACID. Jour. Nutr. 18: 227-232, illus.

(44) POLEY, W.E. and MOXON, A.L. (1938). TOLERANCE LEVELS OF SELENIFEROUS GRAINS IN LAYING RATIONS. Poultry Sci. 17: 72-76, illus.

(45) _____MOXON, A.L. and FRANKE, K.W. (1937). FURTHER STUDIES OF THE EFFECTS OF SELENIUM POISONING ON HATCHABILITY. Poultry Sci. 16: 219-225, illus.

(46) RINGROSE, A.T., NORRIS, L.C. and HEUSER, G.F. (1931). THE OCCURRENCE OF A PELLAGRA-LIKE SYNDROME IN CHICKS. Poultry Sci. 10: 166-177, illus.

(47) SCHUMACHER, A.E. and HEUSER, G.F. (1940). SOME PROPERTIES OF THE ALCOHOL-PRECIPITATE FACTOR WITH FURTHER RESULTS OF ITS EFFECTS ON CHICKS AND HENS. Poultry Sci. 19: 315-320.

(48) STOKSTAD, E.L.R. and MANNING, P.D.V. (1938). THE EFFECT OF RIBOFLAVIN ON THE INCIDENCE OF CURLED TOE PARALYSIS, IN CHICKS. Jour. Nutr. 16: 279-288.

(49) TULLY, W.C. and FRANKE, K.W. (1935). A NEW TOXICANT OCCURRING NATURALLY IN CERTAIN SAMPLES OF PLANT FOODSTUFFS. VI. A STUDY OF THE EFFECT OF AFFECTED GRAINS ON GROWING CHICKS. Poultry Sci. 14: 280-284, illus.

(50) VAN DER HOORN, R., BRANION, B.D. and GRAHAM, W.R., JR. (1935). STUDIES IN THE NUTRITION OF THE CHICK. II. EFFECT OF PURIFICATION OF CASE IN SIMPLIFIED DIET. Poultry Sci. 14: 285-290, illus.

(51) WELCH, HOWARD (1928). GOITER IN FARM ANIMALS. Mont. Agr. Expt. Sta. Bul. 214, 26 pp., illus.

(52) WIESE, A.C., JOHNSON, B.C., ELVEHJEM, C.A. and BART, E.B. (1938). PHOSPHORUS METABOLISM OF CHICKS AFFECTED WITH PEROSIS. Science 88; 383-384.

(53) WILGUS, B.S., GASSNER, F.X., PATTON, A.R. and GUSTAVSON, R.G. (1940). THE GOITROGENICITY OF SOYBEANS. (Abstract of paper) Poultry Sci. 19: 366.

(54) WILGUS, B.S., JR., NOBRIS, L.C. and BEUSER, G.F. (1936). THE ROLE OF CERTAIN INORGANIC ELEMENTS IN THE CAUSE AND PREVENTION OF PEROSIS. Science 84: 252-253.

INDEX

N

R

S